T0226909

Emerging Concepts in Upper Extremity Trauma

Editors

MICHAEL P. LESLIE
SETH D. DODDS

ORTHOPEDIC CLINICS OF NORTH AMERICA

www.orthopedic.theclinics.com

January 2013 • Volume 44 • Number 1

ELSEVIER

1600 John F. Kennedy Blvd. • Suite 1800 • Philadelphia, PA 19103-2899.

http://www.orthopedic.theclinics.com

ORTHOPEDIC CLINICS OF NORTH AMERICA Volume 44, Number 1
January 2013 ISSN 0030-5898, ISBN-13: 978-1-4557-4956-0

Editor: David Parsons

Orthopedic Clinics of North America (ISSN 0030-5898) is published quarterly by Elsevier Inc., 360 Park Avenue South, New York, NY 10010-1710. Months of issue are January, April, July, and October. Business and Editorial Offices: 1600 John F. Kennedy Blvd., Suite 1800, Philadelphia, PA 19103-2899. Customer Service Office: 3251 Riverport Lane, Maryland Heights, MO 63043. Periodicals postage paid at New York, NY and additional mailing offices. Subscription prices are $293.00 per year for (US individuals), $554.00 per year for (US institutions), $347.00 per year (Canadian individuals), $664.00 per year (Canadian institutions), $427.00 per year (international individuals), $664.00 per year (international institutions), $144.00 per year (US students), $208.00 per year (Canadian and international students). Foreign air speed delivery is included in all *Clinics* subscription prices. All prices are subject to change without notice. **POSTMASTER:** Send change of address to *Orthopedic Clinics of North America,* **Elsevier Health Sciences Division, Subscription Customer Service, 3251 Riverport Lane, Maryland Heights, MO 63043. Customer Service (orders, claims, online, change of address): Elsevier Health Sciences Division, Subscription Customer Service, 3251 Riverport Lane, Maryland Heights, MO 63043. Tel: 1-800-654-2452 (U.S. and Canada); 314-447-8871 (outside U.S. and Canada). Fax: 314-447-8029. E-mail: journalscustomerservice-usa@elsevier. com (for print support); journalsonlinesupport-usa@elsevier.com (for online support).**

Reprints. For copies of 100 or more, of articles in this publication, please contact the Commercial Reprints Department, Elsevier Inc., 360 Park Avenue South, New York, NY 10010-1710. Tel.: 212-633-3812; Fax: 212-462-1935; E-mail: reprints@elsevier.com.

Orthopedic Clinics of North America is covered in *MEDLINE/PubMed (Index Medicus), Cinahl, Excerpta Medica,* and *Cumulative Index to Nursing and Allied Health Literature.*

Printed and bound by CPI Group (UK) Ltd, Croydon, CR0 4YY

Transferred to digital print 2012

Contributors

GUEST EDITORS

MICHAEL P. LESLIE, DO
Assistant Professor of Orthopaedics and
Rehabilitation, Trauma and Reconstruction,
Department of Orthopaedics and
Rehabilitation, Yale University School of
Medicine, New Haven, Connecticut

SETH D. DODDS, MD
Associate Professor, Hand and Upper
Extremity Surgery, Associate Program
Director, Orthopaedic Surgery, Department
of Orthopaedics and Rehabilitation, Yale
University School of Medicine, New Haven,
Connecticut

AUTHORS

NICOLAI B. BAECHER, MD
Resident physician, Department of
Orthopaedic Surgery, Georgetown University
Hospital, Washington, DC

MARK E. BARATZ, MD
Professor and Executive Vice Chairman, Hand
and Upper Extremity Service, Department of
Orthopedic Surgery, Allegheny General Hospital,
Drexel University, Pittsburgh, Pennsylvania

DAPHNE M. BEINGESSNER, MD
Associate Professor, Department of
Orthopaedic Surgery and Sports Medicine,
Harborview Medical Center, University of
Washington, Seattle, Washington

SETH D. DODDS, MD
Associate Professor, Hand and Upper Extremity
Surgery, Associate Program Director,
Orthopaedic Surgery, Department of
Orthopaedics and Rehabilitation, Yale University
School of Medicine, New Haven, Connecticut

SCOTT G. EDWARDS, MD
Center for Hand and Elbow Specialists,
Associate Professor, Department of
Orthopaedic Surgery, Georgetown University
Hospital, Washington, DC

THOMAS FISHLER, MD
Clinical Instructor, Department of
Orthopaedics and Rehabilitation, Yale
University School of Medicine, New Haven,
Connecticut

BRODY A. FLANAGIN, MD
Department of Orthopaedics and
Rehabilitation, Yale University School of
Medicine, New Haven, Connecticut

DOUGLAS P. HANEL, MD
Professor, Department of Orthopaedics and
Sports Medicine, Harborview Medical Center,
University of Washington, Seattle, Washington

THOMAS HIGGINS, MD
Associate Professor, University Orthopaedic
Center, University of Utah, Salt Lake City, Utah

STEPHEN A. KENNEDY, MD, FRCSC
Fellow, Hand and Microvascular Surgery,
Department of Orthopaedics and Sports
Medicine, University of Washington, Seattle,
Washington

KATIE E. KINDT, BS
Orthopedic Surgery Department, Allegheny
General Hospital, Pittsburgh, Pennsylvania

AMY L. LADD, MD
Department of Orthopaedic Surgery, Stanford
School of Medicine, Redwood City, California

MARK A. LEE, MD
Associate Professor of Orthopaedic Surgery
and Trauma Fellowship Director, Department
of Orthopaedic Surgery, Ellison ACC,
University of California-Davis, Sacramento,
California

MICHAEL P. LESLIE, DO
Assistant Professor of Orthopaedics and
Rehabilitation, Trauma and Reconstruction,
Yale University School of Medicine, New
Haven, Connecticut

ANNA N. MILLER, MD
Assistant Professor, Department of
Orthopaedic Surgery, Wake Forest University
School of Medicine, Winston-Salem,
North Carolina

DAVID RING, MD, PhD
Chief, Orthopaedic Hand and Upper Extremity
Service, Massachusetts General Hospital;
Associate Professor of Orthopaedic Surgery,
Harvard Medical School, Boston, Massachusetts

DAVID ROTHBERG, MD
Clinical Fellow, Orthopaedic Traumatology,
University of California at Davis, Sacramento,
California

PRASAD J. SAWARDEKER, MD, MS
Orthopedic Surgery Department, Allegheny
General Hospital, Pittsburgh, Pennsylvania

ROSIE SENDHER, MD, MHSC, FRCSC
Department of Orthopaedic Surgery,
Stanford School of Medicine,
Redwood City, California

ROBERT J. STEFFNER, MD
Trauma Fellow, Department of
Orthopaedic Surgery, Ellison ACC,
University of California-Davis,
Sacramento, California

JASON P. WEBER, MD
Resident Physician, Department of
Orthopaedic Surgery, Georgetown University
Hospital, Washington, DC

Contents

Scapulothoracic Dissociation 1

Brody A. Flanagin and Michael P. Leslie

> Scapulothoracic dissociation is rare, resulting from high-energy trauma to the shoulder girdle and disruption of the scapulothoracic articulation. The associated musculoskeletal, vascular, and neurologic injuries carry potentially devastating outcomes. Overall outcomes seem to be closely related to the degree of neurologic impairment sustained. However, given the wide spectrum of injury in scapulothoracic dissociation and limited data concerning outcomes, general recommendations regarding the management of this injury have been difficult to discern. This article reviews the current data regarding the evaluation, diagnosis, treatment, and outcomes after scapulothoracic dissociation.

Fractures of the Proximal Humerus 9

David Rothberg and Thomas Higgins

> Proximal humeral fractures are common, with low-energy injuries occurring in the elderly population and less frequent high-energy fractures striking young people. This article discusses the anatomy, clinical evaluation, and treatment of these fractures.

Emerging Concepts in Upper Extremity Trauma: Humeral Shaft Fractures 21

Robert J. Steffner and Mark A. Lee

> Fractures of the humeral shaft are common in low-energy and high-energy trauma, and optimal clinical management remains controversial. Nonsurgical management has been supported as the preferred treatment based on high union rates and minimal functional deficit due to a rich vascular supply from overlying muscle and the wide motion available at the glenohumeral joint. Recent studies of nonoperative management have challenged surgeons' understanding of these fractures and the perception of favorable outcomes. Current considerations support expanded operative indications with traditional open-plate fixation and with the use of minimally invasive techniques, implants, and a reconsideration of intramedullary nailing.

Intra-Articular Distal Humerus Fractures 35

Anna N. Miller and Daphne M. Beingessner

> Distal humeral fractures are relatively rare and complex injuries. With appropriate preoperative planning and execution of surgical technique, good outcomes may be obtained in most patients. Patients should be counseled regarding loss of motion in these injuries, and elderly, osteoporotic patients with extensive comminution should be considered for total elbow arthroplasty as an alternative to open reduction and internal fixation.

The terrible triad of the elbow is a difficult injury with historically poor outcomes. Improved experience, techniques, and implants have advanced to the point where restoration of elbow stability can be expected. Careful attention to each destabilizing element of the injury pattern is essential and places high demands on the surgeon's mastery of the anatomic complexity of the elbow. Technically, the surgeon must bring every skill to bear, as soft tissue techniques, fracture repair, and joint arthroplasty are routinely required to adequately treat these complex constellations of injury.

Monteggia described a fracture of the proximal third of the ulna with anterior dislocation of the radial head from both the proximal radioulnar and radiocapitellar joints. Application of this eponym to all injuries with radiocapitellar subluxation or dislocation has led to some confusion. In addition, there are substantial differences between Monteggia injuries in children and adults. With careful definition, specific subsets of patients may benefit from consideration as a separate type of Monteggia injury.

Unfortunately, the literature has little guidance for revision elbow surgery. This article attempts to supplement what is known in the literature with the author's anecdotal experience. With this article, it is the author's hope that the reader may learn from his or her successes and his or her failures without having to discover them first hand. There is good reason for angst to overcome surgeons looking at radiographs depicting a traumatized proximal ulna or radius. Surgeons know that there is a good chance they will be seeing these patients for a long time.

Complex distal radius fractures are high-energy injuries of the wrist with articular disruption, ligamentous instability, significant comminution, soft tissue injury, and/or neurovascular impairment. The management of these injuries requires a thorough understanding of wrist functional anatomy and familiarity with a wide selection of approach and fixation options. This article reviews an approach that involves structured evaluation, aggressive open soft tissue injury management, early reduction and skeletal stabilization, and a columnar approach to definitive care. Outcome is determined by multiple factors and depends greatly on the soft tissue injury, patient factors, and management and the adequacy of restoration of osseous and ligamentous relationships.

The progressive perilunar instability model described by Mayfield is still used to predict the pattern of injury. Diagnosis of injury and clinical and radiographic findings depend on the pattern of injury. Open procedures are preferred for anatomic reduction after initial closed reduction is performed for acute injuries. A dorsal, volar, or combined dorsal/volar approach may be necessary and is often decided by surgeon preference. Loss of motion and diminished grip strength are common consequences despite appropriate treatment. Successful outcomes depend on time to treatment, open or closed nature of injury, extent of chondral damage, residual instability, and fracture union.

The scaphoid is vitally important for the proper mechanics of wrist function. Its unique morphology from its boat like shape to its retrograde blood supply can present with challenges in the presence of a fracture. Almost completely covered with articular cartilage, this creates precise surface loading demands and intolerance to bony remodeling. Fracture location compounds risk of malunion and non-union. Scaphoid fractures may significantly impair wrist function and activities of daily living, with both individual and economic consequences.

ORTHOPEDIC CLINICS OF NORTH AMERICA

Preface
From the Scapula to the Scaphoid

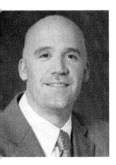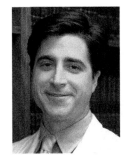

Michael P. Leslie, DO   Seth D. Dodds, MD
Guest Editors

We have challenged an extraordinary group of experts to cut through the typical redundancy of information present and available on upper extremity fracture care. They have more than succeeded in providing succinct articles of the best evidence and experienced opinion.

As editors, we are honored and thankful to have interacted with their carefully composed works. Regardless of whether the reader is a hand surgeon, plastic surgeon, or orthopedic surgeon, we feel this collection offers tremendous opportunity not only to learn but also to understand and digest the emerging concepts of upper extremity trauma.

Michael P. Leslie, DO
Trauma and Reconstruction
Yale University School of Medicine
800 Howard Avenue
New Haven, CT 06520, USA

Department of Orthopaedics and Rehabilitation
Yale University School of Medicine
800 Howard Avenue
P.O. Box 208071
New Haven, CT 06520, USA

Seth D. Dodds, MD
Hand and Upper Extremity Surgery
Orthopaedic Surgery
Department of Orthopaedics and Rehabilitation
Yale University School of Medicine
800 Howard Avenue
P.O. Box 208071
New Haven, CT 06520, USA

E-mail addresses:
michael.leslie@yale.edu (M.P. Leslie)
seth.dodds@yale.edu (S.D. Dodds)

Orthop Clin N Am 44 (2013) ix
http://dx.doi.org/10.1016/j.ocl.2012.09.004
0030-5898/13/$ – see front matter © 2013 Elsevier Inc. All rights reserved.

Scapulothoracic Dissociation

Brody A. Flanagin, MD, Michael P. Leslie, DO*

KEYWORDS

- Scapulothoracic dissociation • Shoulder girdle trauma • Vascular injury • Brachial plexus avulsion

KEY POINTS

- Scapulothoracic dissociation is a rare injury that results from high-energy trauma to the shoulder girdle, leading to disruption of the scapulothoracic articulation.
- The associated injury patterns represent a wide spectrum of musculoskeletal, vascular, and neurologic injuries with potentially devastating outcomes.
- Overall outcomes seem to be closely related to the degree of neurologic impairment sustained at the time of injury. However, given the wide spectrum of injury in scapulothoracic dissociation and limited data concerning outcomes, general recommendations regarding the management of this injury have been difficult to discern.

Scapulothoracic dissociation is a rare, devastating injury resulting from high-energy trauma to the shoulder girdle. Originally described by Oreck and colleagues[1] in 1984, this injury is defined as a traumatic disruption of the scapulothoracic articulation with lateral displacement of the scapula and intact skin. It is believed to result from a high-energy force applied to the shoulder girdle with massive traction to the ipsilateral upper extremity. Scapulothoracic dissociation represents a spectrum of injury that can also include any of the following injuries: Osseous injury to the acromioclavicular (AC) joint, clavicle, and/or sternoclavicular (SC) joint; vascular disruption of the subclavian or axillary vessels; partial or complete avulsion of the brachial plexus; and severe soft-tissue swelling with disruption of the musculature surrounding the shoulder girdle (Fig. 1). As a result, this injury has been characterized as a closed internal forequarter amputation of the upper extremity.[1]

EVALUATION AND DIAGNOSIS

Diagnosis of scapulothoracic dissociation begins with the clinical history and examination. As a result of improved resuscitation protocols and trauma systems, this rare injury pattern is being identified more frequently, making awareness of this clinical entity critical to making the diagnosis.[2] Although scapulothoracic dissociation typically results from high-energy trauma with considerable traction to the involved extremity, confirmation of the exact mechanism may be difficult given an increased chance for associated head trauma. This injury most frequently occurs as a result of motorcycle accidents among reported cases in the literature, but has also been described as sequelae of motor vehicle crashes, falls from heights, and pedestrian versus automobile crashes.[1,3,4] It occurs in both adults and children, and both open and bilateral injuries have been described.[1,3–8] Prompt recognition of this injury pattern is paramount given the concern for life-threatening exsanguination or limb-threatening ischemia from vascular disruption. However, recognition of this exceedingly rare injury pattern can be complicated by many factors, thereby increasing the potential for delayed diagnosis and treatment. Patients with scapulothoracic dissociation have an increased risk for polytrauma given the high amount of energy required to produce this injury.[1,3,4] Associated life-threatening injuries have the potential to distract the emergency

Disclosure: The authors have nothing to disclose.
Department of Orthopaedics and Rehabilitation, Yale University School of Medicine, 800 Howard Avenue, PO Box 208071, New Haven, CT 06520, USA
* Corresponding author. Department of Orthopaedics and Rehabilitation, Yale University School of Medicine, PO Box 208071, New Haven, CT 06520.
E-mail address: Michael.leslie@yale.edu

Orthop Clin N Am 44 (2013) 1–7
http://dx.doi.org/10.1016/j.ocl.2012.09.002

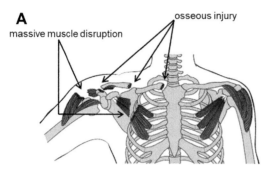
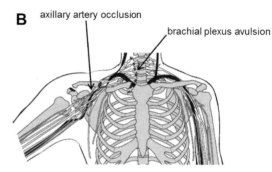

Fig. 1. Scapulothoracic dissociation consists of osseous injury to the AC joint, clavicle, and/or SC joint with disruption of the musculature around the shoulder girdle (*A*) with associated occlusion of the subclavian or axillary artery and partial or complete avulsion of the brachial plexus (*B*).

department physician from a detailed examination of the involved extremity, especially in cases where the patient requires intubation and/or sedation in the prehospital setting.

On clinical examination, severe swelling is typically present around the shoulder as a result of soft-tissue edema and/or hematoma. Complete or partial disruption of the deltoid, pectoralis minor, rhomboids, levator scapulae, trapezius, and latissimus dorsi have all been described as a result of scapulothoracic dissociation.[1,4] Pain, tenderness, and weakness can be present, requiring thorough inspection of the entire shoulder girdle to evaluate for fracture and/or dislocation. Concomitant injuries of the ipsilateral upper extremity as well as other body regions are not uncommon. The appearance and distal perfusion of the involved extremity should be documented. In the patient who is without life-threatening injury and is alert and cooperative, a detailed neurologic examination should be performed to evaluate for brachial plexus injury.

Radiologic evaluation begins with a well-centered chest radiograph. Significant lateral displacement of the scapula is considered pathognomonic for scapulothoracic dissociation (**Fig. 2**). This can be quantified by measuring the scapular index, which is the distance from the midline of the spine to the medial border of the scapula of the affected side divided by that of the noninjured side.[1,9] Normal values lie in the range of 1.07, although 2 small series have reported average scapular indices from 1.29 to as high as 1.50 in patients with scapulothoracic dissociation.[4,9] Because the scapular index requires a well-centered, non-rotated chest radiograph to accurately determine, there is potential for inaccurate measurement. As such, this value should not be considered alone for a diagnosis of scapulothoracic dissociation. Additional radiographs of the scapula as well as computed tomography (CT) scans can be helpful in confirming this diagnosis and are routinely ordered in most level 1 trauma centers caring for patients with significant shoulder

girdle trauma. In addition, associated osseous injuries about the shoulder (AC joint separation, clavicle fracture, SC joint dislocation) occur in association with this injury and appropriate studies should be ordered to evaluate these structures.[3,4]

Diagnosis of vascular injury begins with evaluation of the clinical appearance and distal perfusion of the affected extremity. Pallor, coolness to touch, and mottling can all be present. Pulses should be checked by manual palpation and/or Doppler ultrasonography. Any suspected case of scapulothoracic dissociation necessitates emergent angiography to evaluate for injury to the subclavian, axillary or brachial vessels (**Fig. 3**). Vascular lesions have been reported in 64% to 100% of patients in several small series to date.[1,3,4] The vascular disruption typically results from either intravascular thrombosis or extrinsic arterial compression; death from uncontrolled hemorrhage secondary to vascular disruption is relatively uncommon.[1,3,4,10,11] Furthermore, the

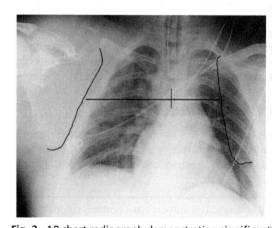

Fig. 2. AP chest radiograph demonstrating significant lateral displacement of the right scapula. The medial border of the scapula has been outlined to highlight the finding. There is also significant soft-tissue swelling about the right shoulder with midshaft clavicle, acromion, and glenoid neck fractures.

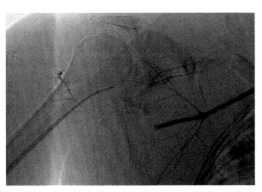

Fig. 3. Angiography demonstrating disruption of the axillary artery.

risk of limb-threatening ischemia of the involved extremity has been reportedly low and may be over-estimated in scapulothoracic dissociation.[2,4,9,11] This is likely owing to a protective effect from the extensive collateral circulation around the shoulder girdle.[12]

Clinical history and physical examination are the cornerstones for evaluation and diagnosis of neurologic injury after scapulothoracic dissociation.[13] This can be complicated by an obtunded or uncooperative patient given the potential for severe injuries to other organ systems. It is critical to perform a complete, detailed neurologic examination to determine whether if the deficit is partial or complete. Damage to the brachial plexus determines the functional prognosis of scapulothoracic dislocations. Complete brachial plexus injury may be associated with preganglionic nerve root avulsions or even rupture of the trunks in the interscalene space.[14] Nerve root avulsions have limited potential for spontaneous recovery, and complete brachial plexus avulsions have been shown to be predictive of poor functional outcome.[4] Weakness of the serratus anterior, rhomboids, and levator scapula are all suggestive of preganglionic injury. Horner's syndrome, consisting of ipsilateral miosis, ptosis, enophthalmos, and anhydrosis, is suggestive of a preganglionic lesion at T1. Lower extremity examination may show evidence of clonus or spasticity, which is suggestive of a cord injury (ie, upper motor neuron).

Rorabeck and Harris[15] originally described 4 prerequisites for establishing an irreversible prognosis for complete brachial plexus injuries: (1) The absence of any clinical recovery; (2) 3 or more pseudomeningoceles on myelography; (3) the absence of voluntary action potentials on repeated electromyographic examinations of C5 to T1; and (4) positive histamine tests in the C5 to T1 territory. CT myelography and magnetic resonance imaging may be considered as a screening

tool for nerve root avulsion, particularly in patients with multilevel lesions. Magnetic resonance imaging generally allows for better imaging of the soft tissues and may be helpful for determining the presence of a pseudomeningocele, which has been strongly correlated with avulsion of the corresponding nerve root.[16] However, 1 study has shown that either magnetic resonance imaging or CT myelography can be used to detect cervical root avulsion with 93% sensitivity in patients with traumatic brachial plexus injuries.[17,18] In cases of complete brachial plexus injury, CT myelography has been suggested as soon as the third week after injury to assess the possibility nerve grafting from an intact root.[14] In the case of incomplete paralysis, neurophysiologic testing may be used to assess trapezius and serratus anterior function, which can assist in planning tendon transfers and soft tissue reconstruction.

Electrodiagnostic studies can be a useful diagnostic aid to determine the involved nerve roots in a patient with a brachial plexus injury. These studies are best delayed until approximately 3 to 4 weeks after injury to best evaluate for complete denervation.[13] Electromyography (EMG) of the deep posterior cervical musculature can be of great value in determining whether the lesion is preganglionic or postganglionic. This determination is made through EMG of the erector spinae, which are innervated by posterior branches of the spinal nerves that exit the root between the spinal cord and the sympathetic ganglion.[13] When there is denervation of the muscles innervated by the plexus that does not include deep posterior cervical musculature, the lesion is presumed to be postganglionic in nature. The combination of clinical examination, upper limb EMG, and paraspinal EMG have been shown to be predictive of the site of the lesion in 80% of patients with either a preganglionic or postganglionic injury and in 67% of patients with a combined injury.

Two main classification systems have been proposed for scapulothoracic dissociation. Damschen and colleagues[10] first proposed a logical system in 1997 to allow for improved clinical decision making regarding diagnosis and management. This was modified in 2004 by Zelle and colleagues[4] in a study on the long-term functional outcome following scapulothoracic dissociation, which differentiates between patients with complete and incomplete brachial plexus avulsion (**Table 1**). A type 1 injury involves musculoskeletal injury alone, whereas type 2A or B adds vascular compromise or incomplete neurologic impairment, respectively. A type 3 pattern consists of musculoskeletal injury with both vascular injury and incomplete neurologic impairment, whereas a type 4

Table 1
Classification scheme for scapulothoracic dissociation according to Zelle et al

Type	Clinical Findings
1	Musculoskeletal injury alone
2A	Musculoskeletal injury with vascular disruption
2B	Musculoskeletal injury with incomplete neurologic injury
3	Musculoskeletal injury with vascular disruption and incomplete neurologic injury
4	Musculoskeletal injury with complete neurologic injury

Data from Ebraheim NA, An HS, Jackson WT, et al. Scapulothoracic dissociation. J Bone Joint Surg Am 1988;70: 428–32.

includes a musculoskeletal injury with complete brachial plexus avulsion. This classification scheme reflects their finding that long-term functional outcomes in their cohort of patients correlated poorly with the classification system proposed by Damschen and colleagues,[19] and that complete brachial plexus avulsion remains the most predictive parameter for poor functional recovery.

TREATMENT

Owing to the rarity, complexity, and variability of the injury pattern seen in scapulothoracic dissociation widely accepted treatment guidelines have not been established. Scapulothoracic dissociation was first described by Oreck and colleagues[1] in 1984, suggesting that most patients before this time expired in the acute time frame after injury, presumably from exsanguination or injuries to other organ systems. As a result of improved trauma care and resuscitation protocols, this rare injury pattern is being identified more frequently.[2] Because the majority of patients have associated traumatic injuries to other organ systems, primary treatment focuses on stabilization and resuscitation according to advanced trauma life support protocols.[1,3,4,10] Once a presumed scapulothoracic dissociation has been identified, further management depends on the severity of any associated injuries as well as the neurologic and hemodynamic status of the patient.

All cases of suspected scapulothoracic dissociation warrant emergent angiography to rule out injury to the subclavian, axillary, or brachial vessels. This is critical to avoid either uncontrolled hemorrhage or prolonged ischemia of the involved extremity.

Emergent exploration and vascular repair is indicated for patients with life-threatening hemorrhage or limb-threatening ischemia. Death from uncontrolled hemorrhage secondary to vascular disruption seems to be uncommon based on reported series in the literature.[1,3,4,10,11] Defining limb-threatening ischemia can be extremely difficult in scapulothoracic dissociation, because most patients have a cool, pulseless extremity.[1–3,11] This is complicated by the fact that many of these patients experience some degree of hypovolemic shock with associated peripheral vasoconstriction. Although some consider absent pulses as suggestive of critical ischemia to the involved extremity, Sampson and colleagues[11] suggested cool temperature and blue mottled discoloration of the affected arm are more indicative of limb-threatening ischemia than pulselessness.[1] When a nonviable extremity is present it has been suggested that vascular repair should be performed within 4 to 6 hours after injury.[10] Interposition grafting with either autologous saphenous vein or polytetraflourorethylene have been described.[11,20] Fasciotomies of the involved extremity may be warranted as well if there is concern for compartment syndrome in an otherwise viable extremity. Based on reported cases in the literature it seems that the risk of limb-threatening ischemia is low, and some authors have even suggested a conservative approach for hemodynamically stable patients with vascular injuries.[2,4,9,11] This is likely owing to a protective effect from the extensive collateral circulation around the shoulder girdle.[12]

Given the broad spectrum of injuries present in scapulothoracic dissociation, stabilization of musculoskeletal injuries should be carried out on an individual basis (**Fig. 4**). A decision regarding bony stabilization and the timing thereof should take into account any associated neurovascular

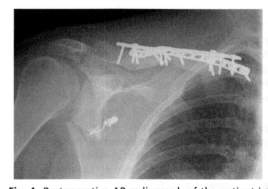

Fig. 4. Postoperative AP radiograph of the patient in **Fig. 1** showing reduction and stabilization of the displaced midshaft clavicle fracture with stacked plating. The acromion and glenoid neck fractures were treated nonoperatively.

njuries requiring repair and any further necessary reconstructive procedures of the involved extremity. Scapulothoracic dissociation is frequently associated with either an SC joint dislocation, displaced clavicle fracture, or AC joint separation.[1,3,4] Patients with musculoskeletal injury alone can be treated with orthopedic stabilization and rehabilitation. Early and appropriate soft tissue coverage should be considered for open injuries.[21] Some authors have suggested application of the principles of the superior shoulder suspensory complex as described by Goss in determining the need for fixation of bony injuries involving the shoulder girdle.[16,21,22] The superior shoulder suspensory complex is a bone and soft-tissue ring composed of the glenoid, distal clavicle, acromion, AC joint, and coracoclavicular ligaments, along with their supporting soft-tissue structures.[22] Although individual disruptions do not typically cause significant compromise of the integrity of the complex, double disruptions are thought to be unstable and can lead to adverse long-term consequences in terms of healing and function if not treated appropriately.[22] Restoring some degree of stability to the shoulder girdle may also offer protection of the injured vessels after vascular repair and support early rehabilitation if an above-elbow amputation is required.[21,22] Clements and Reisser[20] have suggested that stabilization of any orthopedic injuries should be performed before vascular repair in order to determine the appropriate size of the interposition graft. Nonoperative management has been suggested for patients without limb-threatening ischemia to the affected extremity and complete neurologic injury.[10]

The treatment of neurologic injury after scapulothoracic dissociation is determined by the location and severity of the injury. Restoration of elbow flexion is the first priority, followed by shoulder stabilization and adduction of the arm against the chest.[14,16] Final efforts are directed at restoring C6 to C7 sensation and, if possible, wrist extension and finger flexion.[16] Treatment options for brachial plexus lesions include microsurgical nerve repair, nerve grafting, neurotization, tendon transfers, and amputation. Differentiating a preganglionic from a postganglionic lesion determines prognosis and thereby facilitates appropriate surgical planning. If a postganglionic lesion is diagnosed in an otherwise salvageable extremity, nerve repair or grafting can be performed. Nerve repair is chosen when the nerve ends may be sutured together without undue tension, although grafting is indicated when the distance between the 2 stumps does not allow tension-free reapproximation. If a diagnosis of preganglionic lesion is made in the setting of an otherwise salvageable limb or if nerve grafting is unsuccessful, the potential for recovery

is minimal and one may proceed directly to neurotization.[16] In this procedure, an uninjured, less critical nerve is separated from its native muscular insertion and then coupled directly, or via free grafts, to the distal stump of a nonfunctioning nerve. Better results for restoration of elbow flexion have been attained with intercostal to musculocutaneous transfers, whereas spinal accessory to suprascapular transfers seem to have the best outcomes for return ofshoulderabduction.[23–25] Although muscle transfers are well-described for injuries and paralytic conditions in the pediatric population, there are no series in the literature reviewing the functional outcomes of muscle transfers after scapulothoracic dissociation in adult patients with a flail extremity.

Regarding the timing of surgery, it has been suggested that patients who require repair of a vascular injury should also undergo exploration of the brachial plexus to determine the degree of injury.[9] If the brachial plexus seems reparable (ie, midsubstance rupture but no evidence of root avulsion from the spinal cord), some authors recommend nerve repair and/or grafting at the same time as vascular repair.[26] Others have suggested that management of nerve injuries is not emergent, and that nerve reconstruction should preferably be performed within a period of 2 to 6 months from the time of injury with the sole objective of recovering elbow flexion.[14] However, delayed nerve repair/reconstruction can be complicated by scar formation surrounding the nerves of the brachial plexus in patients who have undergone previous vascular repair at the time of injury.[14]

Many authors have recommended above-elbow amputation for patients with a complete brachial plexus avulsion after scapulothoracic dissociation.[1,3,9,10,20,27] A complete brachial plexopathy results in a flail extremity with limited potential for functional recovery that makes independent positioning of the hand in space difficult or impossible. In addition, the spectrum of injury in scapulothoracic dissociation can mimic that of a severe crush injury, thereby increasing the risk for myoglobinuria, hyperkalemia, and late vascular thrombosis. Early amputation can minimize the chance of these complications, especially in patients with severe associated injuries with other organ systems.[16,21] Rorabeck[28] demonstrated that patients with complete brachial plexus injuries who underwent above-elbow amputation within the first year of injury demonstrated earlier to return to work and compliance with their prosthesis. Patients who do choose amputation require a multidisciplinary approach utilizing multiple different care providers to optimize their rehabilitation. Nevertheless, many patients and their families refuse upper extremity amputation, even in the face of a flail extremity.[3,20,27] Yeoman and Seddon[29] recommended combined glenohumeral arthrodesis and above-elbow amputation in patients with a complete brachial plexopathy and flail extremity. They felt it improved the overall function and cosmesis of the affected extremity provided the patient was compliant with wearing a prosthesis. However, this recommendation was based on a small series of patients and it remains unclear whether patients with complete brachial plexus injury and a flail extremity benefit from concomitant shoulder arthrodesis over above-elbow amputation alone.[14,28–30]

OUTCOMES

Previously published reports suggest the mortality rate of scapulothoracic dissociation is roughly 11%.[3] However, it is likely that the overall mortality rate with scapulothoracic dissociation is actually higher and that some patients die from associated injuries in the prehospital setting. There are currently no long-term studies detailing outcomes of fixation of associated musculoskeletal injuries. Although much of the literature has focused on diagnosis and treatment of life-threatening hemorrhage and limb-threatening ischemia in the acute time frame after injury, it has been shown that these complications are relatively uncommon and overall outcomes related to vascular injury are good.[1–4,9–11] This is believed to be owing to a protective effect from the extensive collateral circulation around the shoulder girdle.[12]

Although the impact of vascular injuries on the long-term functional recovery seems to be limited, it has long been speculated that the long-term functional outcome is frequently poor and closely associated with the extent of neurologic injury.[1,3,10,11,14,16,21,27] Riess and colleagues[31] recently reported that patients with a brachial plexus injury in association with scapulothoracic dissociation experienced significantly worse short and long-term functional outcomes over those with an isolated brachial plexus injury alone after blunt trauma. This principle is supported by the fact that functional recovery after complete brachial plexus avulsion is negligible and generally results in a flail, anesthetic upper extremity.[16] This has long been the driving force for recommendation of primary above-elbow amputation in patients with complete brachial plexus avulsions after scapulothoracic dissociation. Reports of nerve reconstruction for complete plexus avulsions are limited in success and, at best, result in restoration of weak elbow flexion and shoulder stability.[14] Zelle and colleagues[3] recently reported the only results in the literature to date documenting long-term

functional outcome in a series of 25 patients after scapulothoracic dissociation. Patients with a complete brachial plexus avulsion had significantly lower scores on the Short-Form 36-Item Health Survey scales and the Subjective Shoulder Rating System at an average follow-up of 12.6 years.[4] It has also been demonstrated in another small series that patients with complete brachial plexus injuries who underwent above-elbow amputation within the first year of injury demonstrated earlier to return to work and compliance with their prosthesis.[28] It would seem, based on the limited data available, that the best long-term functional outcomes in patients with a complete brachial plexus injury are achieved by early above-elbow amputation and immediate postoperative fitting.

SUMMARY

Scapulothoracic dissociation represents occurs as a result of high-energy trauma to the shoulder girdle with massive traction applied to the ipsilateral upper extremity, resulting in disruption of the scapulothoracic articulation with lateral displacement of the scapula and intact skin. This injury is commonly associated with osseous injury to the AC joint, clavicle, and/or SC joint; vascular disruption of the subclavian or axillary vessels; partial or complete avulsion of the brachial plexus; and severe soft-tissue swelling with disruption of the musculature surrounding the shoulder girdle. These patients frequently have associated polytrauma given the high amount of energy required to produce this injury. As a result of improved resuscitation protocols and trauma systems, this rare injury pattern is being identified more frequently, making awareness of this clinical entity critical to making the diagnosis.

Our understanding of this injury is based primarily on small case series and individual case reports. Timely recognition and treatment of any neurovascular injury is critical. Outcomes related to vascular disruption seem to be good, although the extent of damage to the brachial plexus determines the functional prognosis after scapulothoracic dissociation. Complete brachial plexus avulsions generally result in a flail upper extremity with minimal potential for recovery and a poor functional outcome. Early above-elbow amputation and immediate prosthetic fitting has been recommended for patients willing to undergo this procedure, because this approach seems to result in better functional outcomes, earlier return to work, and improved compliance with the use of a prosthesis. More studies are needed to better define overall recommendations regarding the management of patients after scapulothoracic dissociation.

REFERENCES

1. Oreck SL, Burgess A, Levine AM. Traumatic lateral displacement of the scapula: a radiographic sign of neurovascular disruption. J Bone Joint Surg Am 1984;66:758–63.

2. Johansen K, Sangeorzan B, Copass MK. Traumatic scapulothoracic dissociation: case report. J Trauma 1991;31:147–9.

3. Ebraheim NA, An HS, Jackson WT, et al. Scapulothoracic dissociation. J Bone Joint Surg Am 1988; 70:428–32.

4. Zelle BA, Pape HC, Gerich TG, et al. Functional outcome following scapulothoracic dissociation. J Bone Joint Surg Am 2004;86:2–8.

5. Lovejoy J, Ganey TM, Ogden JA. Scapulothoracic dissociation secondary to major shoulder trauma. J Pediatr Orthop B 2009;18:131–4.

6. An HS, Vonderbrink JP, Ebraheim NA, et al. Open scapulothoracic dissociation with intact neurovascular status in a child. J Orthop Trauma 1988;2:36–8.

7. Fischer PJ II, Kent RB III. Open scapulothoracic dissociation. South Med J 2001;94:383–6.

8. Lange RH, Noel SH. Traumatic lateral scapular displacement: an expanded spectrum of associated neurovascular injury. J Orthop Trauma 1993;7:361–6.

9. Kelbel JM, Jardon OM, Huurman WW. Scapulothoracic dissociation. A case report. Clin Orthop Relat Res 1986;209:210–4.

10. Damschen DD, Cogbill TH, Siegel MJ. Scapulothoracic dissociation caused by blunt trauma. J Trauma 1997;42:537–40.

11. Sampson LN, Britton JC, Eldrup-Jorgensen J, et al. The neurovascular outcome of scapulothoracic dissociation. J Vasc Surg 1993;17:1083–8.

12. Levin PM, Rich NM, Hutton JE Jr. Collateral circulation in arterial injuries. Arch Surg 1971;102:392–9.

13. Leffert RD. Clinical diagnosis, testing, and electromyographic study in brachial plexus traction injuries. Clin Orthop Relat Res 1988;237:24–31.

14. Masmejean EH, Asfazadourian H, Alnot JY. Brachial plexus injuries in scapulothoracic dissociation. J Hand Surg Br 2000;25:336–40.

15. Rorabeck CH, Harris WR. Factors affecting the prognosis of brachial plexus injuries. J Bone Joint Surg Br 1981;63:404–7.

16. Brucker PU, Gruen GS, Kaufmann RA. Scapulothoracic dissociation: evaluation and management. Injury 2005;36:1147–55.

17. Doi K, Otsuka K, Okamoto Y, et al. Cervical nerve root avulsion in brachial plexus injuries: magnetic resonance imaging classification and comparison with myelography and computerized tomography myelography. J Neurosurg 2002;96:277–84.

18. Balakrishnan G, Kadadi BK. Clinical examination versus routine and paraspinal electromyographic studies in predicting the site of lesion in brachial plexus injury. J Hand Surg Am 2004;29:140–3.

19. Damschen DD, Cogbill TH, Siegel MJ. Scapulothoracic dissociation caused by blunt trauma. J Trauma 1997;42:537–40.

20. Clements RH, Reisser JR. Scapulothoracic dissociation: a devastating injury. J Trauma 1996;40:146–9.

21. Althausen PL, Lee MA, Finkemeier CG. Scapulothoracic dissociation: diagnosis and treatment. Clin Orthop Relat Res 2003;416:237–44.

22. Goss TP. Double disruptions of the superior shoulder suspensory complex. J Orthop Trauma 1993;7:99–106.

23. Songcharoen P, Mahaisavariya B, Chotigavanich C. Spinal accessory neurotization for restoration of elbow flexion in avulsion injuries of the brachial plexus. J Hand Surg Am 1996;21:387–90.

24. Waikakul S, Wongtragul S, Vanadurongwan V. Restoration of elbow flexion in brachial plexus avulsion injury: comparing spinal accessory nerve transfer with intercostal nerve transfer. J Hand Surg Am 1999;24:571–7.

25. Merrell GA, Barrie KA, Katz DL, et al. Results of nerve transfer techniques for restoration of shoulder and elbow function in the context of a meta-analysis of the English literature. J Hand Surg Am 2001;26: 303–14.

26. Ebraheim NA, Pearlstein SR, Savolaine ER, et al. Scapulothoracic dissociation (closed avulsion of the scapula, subclavian artery, and brachial plexus): a newly recognized variant, a new classification, and a review of the literature and treatment options. J Orthop Trauma 1987;1:18–23.

27. Goldstein LJ, Watson JM. Traumatic scapulothoracic dissociation: case report and literature review. J Trauma 2000;48:533–5.

28. Rorabeck CH. The management of the flail upper extremity in brachial plexus injuries. J Trauma 1980;20:491–3.

29. Yeoman PM, Seddon HJ. Brachial plexus injuries: treatment of the flail arm. J Bone Joint Surg Br 1961;43:493–500.

30. Bedi A, Miller B, Jebson PJ. Combined glenohumeral arthrodesis and above elbow amputation for the flail limb following a complete posttraumatic brachial plexus injury. Tech Hand Up Extrem Surg 2005;9:113–9.

31. Riess KP, Cogbill TH, Patel NY, et al. Brachial plexus injury: long-term functional outcome is determined by associated scapulothoracic dissociation. J Trauma 2007;63:1021–5.

Fractures of the Proximal Humerus

David Rothberg, MD[a],*, Thomas Higgins, MD[b]

KEYWORDS

- Proximal humerus fracture • Neer classification • Fibular strut • Shoulder arthroplasty

KEY POINTS

- Proximal humeral fractures are common.
- Classification systems have evolved to develop treatment guidelines.
- Bone quality must be considered for treatment.
- Surgical stabilization may require augmentation.
- Arthroplasty must be considered especially in the elderly.

INTRODUCTION

Proximal humeral fractures are common, with low-energy injuries occurring in the elderly population and less frequent higher-energy fractures striking young people. The decision to pursue operative or nonoperative treatment is driven by the functional goals and the degree of displacement of the proximal humeral anatomic parts. Operative management is based on the ability to obtain and maintain reduction, vascularity of the articular segment, quality of soft-tissue attachments, and bone porosity. Despite much study, the optimal treatment of significantly displaced fracture patterns remains controversial.

EPIDEMIOLOGY

Fractures of the proximal humerus are common, occurring in 4% of the population. They are most commonly attributed to low-energy falls, with a smaller subset of high-energy injuries affecting a younger population, but overall incidence increases as bone mineral density decreases. Proximal humeral fractures are the third most common osteoporotic extremity fracture after hip fractures and distal radius fractures.[1] Greater than 70% of these fractures occur in patients older than 60 years, with a 4:1 female/male ratio and an incidence steadily increasing after the age of 40 years.

Independent risk factors for proximal humeral fractures include a recent decline in health status, insulin-dependent diabetes mellitus, infrequent walking, indicators of neuromuscular weakness, diminished femoral neck bone density, height/weight loss, previous falls, impaired balance, and maternal history of hip fractures.[2] In a 3-decade population-based study of osteoporotic proximal humeral fractures, Palvanen and colleagues[3] found that the incidence in patients older than 60 years increased by 13.7% per year of age. When adjusted for age, the incidence of proximal humeral fracture increased in women by 243% and in men by 153%. This increase was attributed to the expanding elderly population as well as the increasing incidence in the risk factors mentioned previously. Based on the observed trends, they calculated that the incidence of proximal humeral fractures would triple by 2030.

No disclosures relevant to this article.
[a] Orthopaedic Traumatology, University of California at Davis, 4860 Y Street, Suite 3800, Sacramento, CA 95817, USA; [b] University Orthopaedic Center, University of Utah, 590 Wakara Way, Salt Lake City, UT 84108, USA
* Corresponding author.
E-mail address: David.rothberg@ucdmc.ucdavis.edu

Orthop Clin N Am 44 (2013) 9–19
http://dx.doi.org/10.1016/j.ocl.2012.08.004
0030-5898/13/$ – see front matter © 2013 Elsevier Inc. All rights reserved.

ANATOMY

The 4 basic osseous structures that serve as the basis for restoration of normal anatomy after reduction are the articular surface proximal to the anatomic neck, greater tuberosity, lesser tuberosity, and humeral shaft. The articular segment has no muscular attachments. The supraspinatus, infraspinatus, and teres minor muscles attach to the greater tuberosity; the subscapularis attaches to the lesser tuberosity; and the deltoid, pectoralis major, teres major, and latissimus dorsi attach to the humeral shaft. The normal osseous relationships define goals for reduction. In the coronal plane the humeral head is inclined to the shaft by a neck shaft angle of 130° to 150°. The humeral head center is offset medially 4 to 14 mm from the center of the shaft and −2 to 10 mm posteriorly. The most proximal aspect of the humeral head articular surface is 8 mm from the tip of the greater tuberosity. In the sagittal plane, the humeral head is retroverted to the shaft by 0° to 55°.

Given the propensity for avascular necrosis of the humeral head after proximal humeral fracture, the perfusion of this area has been the focus of much study. The primary vascular supply to the humeral head is through the anterior humeral circumflex artery. In a latex injection dissection study, Gerber and colleagues[4] showed the anterior humeral circumflex artery to originate from the axillary artery at 1 cm distal to the pectoralis major, running between the short head of the biceps and the coracobrachialis and reaching the surgical neck of the humerus at the inferior border of the subscapularis. The most important branch, the anterolateral branch, traverses under the long head of the biceps adjacent to the lateral border of the intertubercular groove, entering the head at the transition of the intertubercular groove and the greater tuberosity. Once the vessel penetrates the head, it runs as the arcuate artery, posteromedially within the epiphysis, supplying all but a small portion of the posteroinferior portion of the epiphysis and the adjacent posterior portion of the greater tuberosity. The posterior humeral circumflex artery arises from the axillary artery and perfuses the posteroinferior portion of the epiphysis and the posterior greater tuberosity anastomosing with the anterior humeral circumflex artery in the region of the joint capsule and greater tuberosity.[4]

Further study into the humeral head blood supply after fracture shows that, although the anterior humeral circumflex artery is the main blood supply, the head may stay perfused despite its frequent disruption. The anterior humeral circumflex artery is disrupted in 80% of fractures, whereas the posterior humeral circumflex is intact in 85%. In magnetic resonance imaging angiography studies, Hettrich and colleagues[5] showed that the posterior humeral circumflex artery may perfuse up to 64% of the humeral head, which explains the clinical finding of perfusion after fracture. Studies using different evaluation tools have shown contradicting findings, but there seems to be fracture-specific predictors of humeral head ischemia. Hertel and colleagues[6] showed that humeral head ischemia could be predicted with a 97% positive predictive value when the metaphyseal head extension length was less than 8 mm, when there was disruption of the medial hinge between the humeral head and shaft, and when there was an anatomic neck component (**Fig. 1**).

EVALUATION
Mechanism of Injury

History reveals one or a combination of mechanisms occurring to produce a fracture of the proximal humerus: (1) direct blows in the setting of high-energy trauma, (2) falls from standing height, (3) axial loads, (4) excessive internal rotation and adduction forces.

Clinical Evaluation

After evaluation for concomitant upper extremity, neck, and chest wall injuries, as may be present in high-energy trauma, a thorough neurovascular examination is performed. Motor evaluation of the brachial plexus innervation is performed by evaluating the deltoid, biceps, triceps, and wrist flexors/extensors and hand intrinsics motor examination. So-called pseudoparalysis, thought to be secondary to swelling and pain, may make this examination difficult, and the presence of deltoid function does not always rule out an axillary nerve injury. Axillary nerve neuropraxia is the most common deficit in the setting of proximal humeral fracture. Sensation is evaluated through dermatomal light touch examination, and careful evaluation of perfusion to the hand should be documented as well.

Associated Injury

Vascular injury to the axillary artery, although rare, may have devastating consequences if not identified. It may present as obvious acute ischemia or subtly as increasing pain, loss of sensation, and axillary swelling with ecchymosis. The axillary artery is at risk as it crosses medial to the head and surgical neck of the humerus and may be damaged by direct laceration from displaced fracture fragments or by traction to the upper

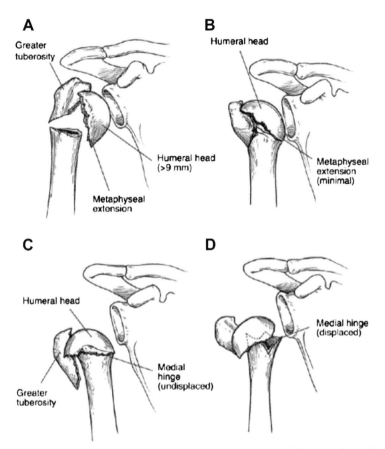

Fig. 1. Hertel's radiographic criteria. Metaphyseal extension is the measured distance from the head–neck junction to the inferior extent of the medial cortex. (*A*) Metaphyseal extension greater than 8 mm. (*B*) Metaphyseal extension less than 8 mm. The medial hinge is evaluated at the medial calcar. (*C*) Intact medial hinge. (*D*) Medial hinge displaced greater than 2 mm. (*Adapted from* Hertel R, Hempfing A, Stiehler M, et al. Predictors of the humeral head ischemia after intracapsular fracture of the proximal humerus. J Shoulder Elbow Surg 2004; 13:427–33; with permission.)

extremity. Prompt arteriography and subsequent repair is necessary and may be timed with fracture fixation to prevent further injury.

A significant factor in the outcome of proximal humeral fractures is associated injury to the brachial plexus. Neurologic injury associated with proximal humeral fracture is most common in the axillary nerve distribution. Large fracture fragment displacement with associated hematoma development and older age show increasing incidences of axillary nerve injury. Complete evaluation of neurologic injury is often difficult secondary to pain and swelling associated with the fracture. Most associated neurologic injuries partially or completely resolve within 4 months.

Rotator cuff injury is common after proximal humeral fractures with rates of 29% to 40%.[7] The severity of the tear correlates with increasing Neer and AO-OTA (AO-Orthopaedic Trauma Association) classification and subsequent displacement of the greater tuberosity fragment.[7] The role of the rotator cuff tear in the functional recovery of proximal humeral fractures is incompletely defined. Two reports on the functional outcome in conservatively treated proximal humeral fractures with rotator cuff tears are inconclusive with respect to outcome; therefore, advanced imaging for complete evaluation of the rotator cuff in the setting of proximal humeral fracture cannot be recommended at this time.

Radiographic Evaluation

Radiographic evaluation with 3 views of the shoulder is critical to successful diagnosis, classification, and treatment. Anteroposterior (AP), axillary lateral, and scapular Y views of the shoulder are obtained in a trauma series. The true AP view (Grashey view) shows the articular surface and defines the main fracture line between the head, neck and shaft, the head/neck shaft angle, the glenohumeral relationship, and the varus/valgus displacement in the coronal plane. The axillary lateral view defines the relationship of the humeral head with respect to the glenoid in the axial plane, allowing evaluation of glenohumeral dislocation as well as AP translation of the head to the shaft. The glenoid should be well visualized, and scapular pathologic findings may be identified with proximal humeral fractures, particularly in high-energy injuries. The scapular Y view gives information on the displacement of the humeral head relative to the shaft in the sagittal plane, as well as greater tuberosity displacement, but the superimposed scapula may obscure fracture anatomy (**Fig. 2**).

The major fracture fragment relationships may not be clearly defined in multifragmentary fracture patterns. The indications for computed tomographic (CT) examination vary widely but include cases in which fracture overlap and low-quality axillary lateral views may obscure relevant pathoanatomy. CT axial cuts show the glenohumeral relationship when an axillary lateral is unobtainable. Both 2-dimensional cuts and 3-dimensional reconstructions demonstrate major fracture fragment relationships better than plain radiography. CT is also useful when humeral head involvement is suspected, such as humeral head impaction or head-splitting fractures.

CLASSIFICATION

The Neer classification system is based on fragment displacement rather than fracture lines and depicts the pathoanatomy of the soft tissues as well as the bone (**Fig. 3**).[8] The 4 segments are Codman major fragments, including the anatomic neck, surgical neck, and greater and lesser tuberosities. The fracture classification comprises 18 fracture patterns in 4 categories based on number and displacement of segments, called parts. A part is defined as displacement of a fragment by at least 1 cm or rotation of at least 45°. Articular surface and head-splitting fractures are 2 subcategories that do not fit neatly in these categorizations.

A proximal humeral fracture that does not have displacement of a single part, regardless of fracture lines, is considered a 1-part fracture. These fractures are held together by soft-tissue attachments or are minimally affected.

Two-Part Fractures

Anatomic neck 2-part fractures are rare and consist of the articular surface rotated or displaced into varus as the tuberosities prevent valgus displacement. Surgical neck 2-part fractures occur with the shaft displaced anteriorly and rotated inwardly from the articular surface and tuberosities. Impacted 2-part fractures usually are displaced apex anterior with a periosteal hinge posteriorly. Nonimpacted 2-part surgical neck fractures have shaft displacement anteromedially, with the articular fragment in neutral rotation. Comminuted 2-part surgical neck fractures usually have an anteromedially displaced shaft fragment, with the head in neutral rotation. Greater tuberosity 2-part fractures tend to occur after anterior glenohumeral dislocations, and the tuberosity is displaced superior and posterior along the path of the superior rotator cuff muscles. Lesser tuberosity 2-part fractures tend to occur after forceful muscle

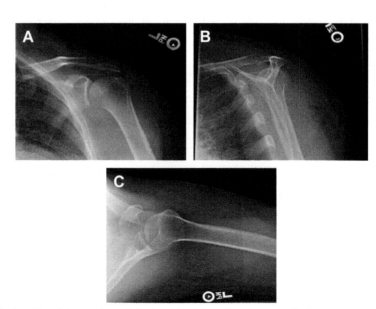

Fig. 2. (*A*) AP left shoulder, (*B*) scapular Y left shoulder, (*C*) axillary lateral left shoulder.

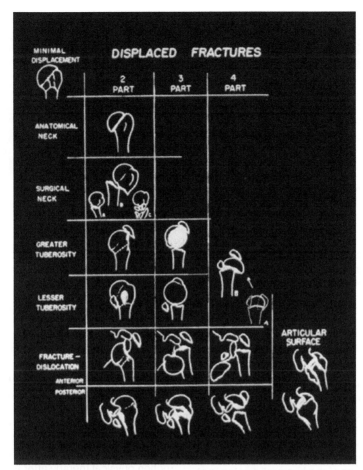

Fig. 3. Neer classification. (*From* Neer CS. Four-segment classification of proximal humeral fractures: purpose and reliable use. J Shoulder Elbow Surg 2002;11(4):389; with permission.)

contraction of the subscapularis, as in seizures, and the tuberosity displaces medially.

Three-Part Fractures

When 3-part fractures occur, 1 tuberosity remains attached to the articular surface and rotates around a nonimpacted surgical neck fragment. When the lesser tuberosity is displaced, the head rotates externally. When the greater tuberosity is displaced, the head rotates internally.

Four-Part Fractures

Four-part fractures occur in 2 patterns, valgus impacted 4-part fractures and lateral displacement fracture dislocations. Neer described the valgus impacted 4-part fracture as a borderline lesion with less lateral displacement than a true 4-part fracture.[8] In the valgus impacted fracture the tuberosities displace away from the articular segment, allowing it to impact on the shaft. The articular segment rotates at least 45° but does not displace laterally and may have an intact medial periosteal hinge. In the lateral displacement 4-part fracture, the articular segment displaces allowing for varus deformity (**Fig. 4**). When the articular segment is not in congruity with the glenoid, it is considered a fracture dislocation and may be present in any subcategory but is always present in true 4-part fractures. Fracture dislocations are named according to the direction of displacement of the articular fragment.

The AO-OTA classification system is based on the Neer classification but allows for more expanded subgroupings.[9] It has 3 basic groups containing many subgroups. The expanded subgroupings are meant to place more emphasis on the displacement of 2-part anatomic neck fractures, displacement as it relates to functional compromise or vascular discontinuity and a greater number of subgroupings, for detailed analysis. Type A fractures are unifocal, extraarticular 2-part fractures with intact vascular supply. Type B fractures are bifocal, extraarticular fractures with

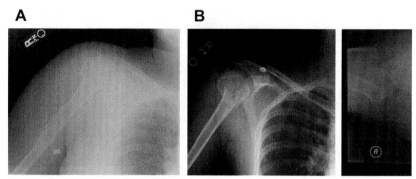

Fig. 4. (*A*) AP radiograph shows a valgus impacted 4-part fracture with an intact medial hinge. (*B*) AP and axillary lateral radiographs show a 4-part fracture dislocation with varus deformity and no contact between the articular piece and the glenoid.

possible injury to the vascular supply. Type C fractures are articular fractures involving the anatomic neck with high likelihood of injury to the osseous blood supply.

TREATMENT
General Considerations: Age/Bone Quality

In addition to fracture pattern and displacement, the physiologic age and bone quality of a patient should be considered to estimate the likelihood of success of internal fixation. Combined cortical thickness is the mean of the medial and lateral cortex width at 2 levels, adjusted for magnification, on an AP radiograph. The first level evaluated is the most proximal aspect of the humeral diaphysis at which the cortices are parallel to each other. The second level is a point 20 mm distal to the first level.[10] A combined cortical thickness of less than 4 mm indicates low bone mineral density. A combined cortical thickness of greater than 4 mm has demonstrated a significantly lower incidence of failure with plate and screw constructs. It is postulated that when the combined cortical thickness is not adequate, alternative methods of treatment including nonoperative management, suture fixation, or arthroplasty must be considered.

General Considerations: Viability of the Articular Segment

As mentioned previously, Hertel and colleagues[6] have elegantly delineated 3 predictors of humeral head ischemia; metaphyseal extension less than 8 mm, loss of medial hinge integrity, and fractures with an anatomic neck component. The outcome of patients with osseous necrosis is generally poor when collapse is present; however, without collapse this is rarely symptomatic. If predictors of ischemia are present, near anatomic reduction must be achieved for a successful outcome. If

the surgeon is unable to restore anatomic alignment, arthroplasty may provide better results.

Nonoperative Treatment

Minimally displaced proximal humeral fractures most commonly occur with a fall from standing height in a woman older than 60 years. They may be classified by the Neer classification as 1-part fractures or by the AO-OTA classification in the groups A, B, or C. The most minimally displaced fractures are type A fractures (76%), with types B and C occurring at older ages (61 vs 69 years). Most patients are treated with a simple sling for 10 to 14 days and supervised active range of motion physical therapy after the sling is removed. Radiographs are taken at 3-week intervals to check for fracture displacement. The vast majority of fractures do not displace significantly, but settling of the surgical neck is common.

In the largest series to date, Gaebler and colleagues[11] retrospectively reviewed 507 minimally displaced proximal humeral fractures in individuals with an average age of 63 years. Age and premorbid condition negatively correlated with outcome and return to activities of daily living although 88% had good to excellent results.

Although nonoperative treatment performs well in nondisplaced and minimally displaced fractures, displaced fractures show diminishing functional results in the more advanced Neer classification groups.[12] These fractures have been traditionally treated with a sling or hanging cast, with no difference between the treatment modalities. Yuksel and colleagues[13] studied the results of nonoperative treatment in 3- and 4-part fractures without articular involvement or head splitting. Of their 18 patients, 33% had valgus impaction, 28% had osseous necrosis, and 16% had nonunion, and these results are consistent with other literature. Those with 3-part fractures performed better on

Constant scores than those with 4-part fractures, with an average Constant score of 61.3 for the cohort. Osseous necrosis and valgus impaction did not significantly affect outcome. Although this study showed higher functional outcomes with younger patients overall, age adjustment shows older patients (age >60 years) perform better with nonoperative management.[13]

Suture Fixation

Although more commonly applied to 2-part tuberosity fractures, suture fixation using transosseous and tension band techniques have been used successfully in 2-, 3- and 4-part valgus impacted fractures.[50] Relying on the strength of the rotator cuff tendons rather than that of the bone, suture techniques may be best suited in patients with less than 4 mm combined cortical thickness.

Transdeltoid and deltopectoral intervals have been used with various suture techniques depending on fracture pattern. Two-part tuberosity fractures use heavy nonabsorbable sutures through the rotator cuff tendons affixed to the humeral shaft through transosseous drill holes. Three- and four-part valgus impacted fractures rely on the reduction of the articular segment to the humeral shaft and suture closure of the rotator interval before a transosseous suture fixation of the tuberosities. Low rates of osseous necrosis and nonunion have been reported with 77% to 100% good to excellent results with these techniques.[14]

Closed Reduction and Percutaneous Pinning

Closed reduction and percutaneous pinning (CRPP) has been primarily indicated for 2-part fractures with minimal comminution and 3- and 4-part valgus impacted fractures with minimal comminution of the tuberosities. The technique is theoretically soft-tissue sparing and may reduce vascular/healing complications associated with extensive dissection. The tenuous purchase of pins would suggest avoiding this procedure in patients with a combined cortical width of less than 4 mm. The safety zone for lateral pin placement is twice the distance from the superior and inferior margins of the humeral head cartilage. For greater tuberosity, the pins should engage the medial cortex at least 2 cm below the humeral head cartilage and the shoulder should be held in external rotation during their placement.[15]

Initial experience with CRPP showed it to be technically demanding, with high complication rates of pin migration, loss of reduction, and pin site infection. These complications have led to technique modifications with terminally threaded pins and external fixation devices with good results in some series.

Open Reduction Internal Fixation (Locked vs Nonlocked)

Conventional nonlocked plating may be appropriate for 2-part surgical neck fractures and 3-part fractures that do not include significant comminution or poor bone quality. Successful conventional plating requires anatomic reduction aided by greater than 3.5 mm of diaphyseal cortex and a lack of metaphyseal comminution.[16] Factors that complicate the use of conventional plating techniques include poor bone quality, comminution, fracture gap, an articular segment associated with the fracture pattern, or an inability to gain screw purchase in the center of the humeral head.[16] The extensive dissection required for reduction and plate fixation may put the head at risk for vascular compromise.

Because fractures of the proximal humerus are more common in the elderly, the mechanical limits of conventional plating are commonly exposed when used in less-than-ideal settings. The high incidence of osteoporosis in those older than 60 years leads to mechanical failure of conventional plate-and-screw constructs when the fracture pattern does not provide axial and angular stability after reduction. Conventional screws may be optimized in osteoporotic bone by placing them parallel to cancellous trabeculae and obtaining purchase in the stronger cortical bone. When the fracture environment does not allow adequate purchase, locked plating constructs provide a mechanical advantage.

The evolution of proximal humeral plate osteosynthesis is similar to that in the distal femur fracture. In both cases, a fairly small articular segment is adjacent to metaphyseal comminution, and locked plating has radically improved the ability to obtain purchase in the articular segment and resist varus cutout. Locked plates provide axial and angular stability by creating a fixed-angle construct that converts sheer to compression at the bone–screw interface (**Fig. 5**A). Fractures with osteoporotic bone, metaphyseal comminution, or fracture gap may benefit from the advantages of locked plate stability to hold reduction and prevent the complications of excessive fracture motion.

The initial enthusiasm in small case series showing less complications and revisions using locked plates for proximal humeral fractures has been tempered. There have been 2 prospective randomized controlled trials comparing locked plate fixation to nonoperative treatment.[17] Olerud

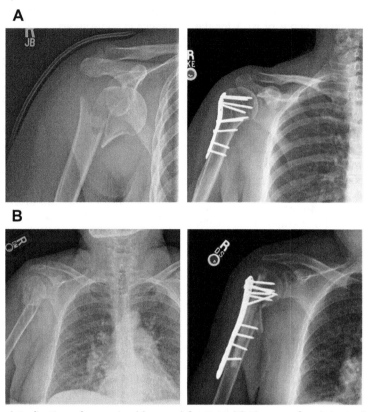

Fig. 5. (*A*) Locked-plate fixation of a proximal humeral fracture. (*B*) The use of an intramedullary fibular strut allograft as a tool to maintain medial reduction of the head.

and colleagues[17] prospectively randomized 3-part fractures in the elderly to locked plates or nonoperative treatment and showed a benefit in functional outcome and health-related quality of life in the locked-plate group in terms of clinical difference but not statistical significance. Thirty percent of the 27 patients who received locked plating needed an additional operation. Twenty-nine percent ultimately demonstrated intra-articular screw penetration, 16% had displacement of a tuberosity, and 10% had osseous necrosis. Fjalestad and colleagues[18] prospectively randomized elderly patients with 3- and 4-part fractures to locked plates or nonoperative treatment. They had 50 patients evenly distributed to each group, showing no significant difference in functional outcome or self-assessment, although radiographic outcomes were significantly better in the locked-plate group. The mean, adjusted Constant score was 74.4 for both groups with a 32% osseous necrosis rate, but 28% of the operative patients had intra-articular screw penetration. There was a higher rate of osseous necrosis in the nonoperative group at 52%. The most recent meta-analysis on locked plating included 514 patients in 12 studies showing a mean Constant score of 74, with an overall complication rate of 49% and a reoperation rate of 14%. The most common complications were varus malunion 16%, osseous necrosis 10%, intra-articular screw perforation 8%, subacromial impingement 6%, and infection 4%.[19]

SURGICAL TECHNIQUE

Surgical approach is most commonly deltopectoral, but a lateral deltoid splitting approach has gained popularity in recent years. Reduction is performed in a stepwise manner, starting with relocation of the head when dislocation is present. Visualization may be obtained with a rotator interval dissection if necessary, being careful to not devitalize the soft-tissue attachments. Reducing the head to the shaft is the next step in valgus impacted fractures and those 3-part fractures with a tuberosity attached to the articular segment. In varus fractures the head is reduced to the shaft after reduction of the tuberosities. Tuberosity reduction may be aided by heavy suture placement at the rotator cuff tendon-to-bone interface.

Fixation with a locked plate is aided by placing the plate and screw appropriately and bringing the articular segment out of a varus position, if present. Residual varus angulation accelerates fracture displacement and superior screw cutout. The plate is placed inferior to the most superior portion of the greater tuberosity to prevent impingement on the acromion and lateral to the bicipital groove to prevent disruption of the humeral head blood supply. Screws should be placed within 5 to 10 mm of the articular surface where the subchondral bone is most dense. The addition of inferomedial calcar supporting screws helps maintain reduction in fractures that have initial varus angulation or medial metaphyseal comminution.

Intramedullary Nail

Intramedullary nails have been used mainly for 2-part surgical neck fractures with good results. Initial series showed significant varus collapse at fracture healing, but with the advent of angular stable nails, collapse rates in one series were similar to those of modern locked plates. Advocates of intramedullary nailing cite the proximal greater tuberosity entry point as beneficial, as it does not violate the proximal humeral blood supply and may decrease rates of osseous necrosis. One prospective analysis of locked plates and intramedullary nails for the treatment of 2-part surgical neck fractures has shown decreased supraspinatus muscle strength in the nail group, increased screw cutout in the plate group, and similar forward elevation and outcomes scores between the groups.[20] When used in 2-, 3-, and 4-part proximal humeral fractures, complication rates have been similar to locked plates with respect to screw cutout, varus collapse with malunion, and revision rates, and outcomes scores have been similar. Fractures that stand out as not being amenable to intramedullary fixation are those with isolated tuberosity fractures or those with unstable or comminuted lateral metaphysis that extend into the nail entry.

Biologic Augmentation

The proximal humerus has been described as a "hen's egg," with decreasing bone mineral density as the geometric center of the head is approached.[89,90] As bone density decreases with age, there is variable but commonly present metaphyseal impaction that may leave a cancellous void and subsequent fracture instability after reduction. Bone substitutes, autograft bone, and allograft bone have been used to fill this void. Intramedullary fibular strut grafts have been used as void fillers, fracture gap and comminution bridges, reduction tools, and a method to achieve better screw purchase in those fractures that have combined cortical widths of less than 4 mm. Using an intramedullary strut significantly increases the initial stiffness and load to failure in a locking plate construct (see **Fig. 5B**). The results of using the fibular intramedullary strut have been promising in some series. Neviaser and colleagues[21] showed a mean Constant score of 87 in thirty-eight 2-, 3-, and 4-part fractures treated with an intramedullary fibular strut graft. One patient lost reduction with varus collapse but did not require further surgery, and one had asymptomatic osseous necrosis and no intra-articular screw penetration or screw cutout. Intramedullary struts may complicate subsequent arthroplasty, as they can obliterate the canal.

Arthroplasty

In fractures in which there is significant articular involvement such as head-splitting fractures and articular impaction fractures, in elderly patients with a fracture that has a high likelihood of vascular insult based on Hertel's criteria, or in fractures in which acceptable alignment and fixation cannot be obtained based on fracture pattern or bone quality, hemiarthroplasty should be considered. The results of hemiarthroplasty are modest, and a recent review of 16 studies with 810 hemiarthroplasties and a mean follow-up of 3.7 years showed that pain relief is universal but function is markedly limited.[22] Mean active forward flexion and abduction were 106° and 92°, respectively. Results are limited by high tuberosity nonunion rates of 11%, heterotopic ossification rates of 8.8%, and humeral head proximal migration rates of 6.8%. The mean Constant score among all studies was 56.6.

Technical factors in the hemiarthroplasty group that correlated significantly with poor outcome were a negative humeral head height variance and positive medial calcar offset. Tuberosity malunion and nonunion also correlate significantly with poor outcome, causing limited motion and subacromial impingement. Ideal positioning of a hemiarthroplasty should mimic the length of the nonoperative limb, with greater tuberosity position approximately 8 mm below the humeral head, the lesser tuberosity anatomically reduced, the head at approximately 30° to 40° of retroversion to the shaft, and less than 5 mm of medial calcar offset.

The complications affecting the outcome of hemiarthroplasty for proximal humeral fracture are related to rotator cuff function. For this reason, reverse shoulder arthroplasty has been introduced into the treatment of the nonreconstructable fractures in elderly patients. Indications for reverse shoulder arthroplasty are elderly patient with a nonreconstructable fracture pattern, massive rotator cuff tear, irreparable tuberosity fracture, comorbidities that prevent tuberosity healing, failed hemiarthroplasty, or chronic fracture. These are summarized as a perceived inability to achieve tuberosity union with a standard hemiarthroplasty. There is not adequate data now to make meaningful conclusions on the outcome. The most common complication of reverse shoulder arthroplasty for fracture is scapular notching (0%–53%), followed by tuberosity malunion/nonunion (0%–46%) and heterotopic ossification (0%–88%). There is only 1 study directly comparing hemiarthroplasty with reverse shoulder arthroplasty for fracture. Gallinet and colleagues[23] showed increased active forward elevation (98° vs 54°) and increased Constant score (53 vs 39) but decreased external rotation (9° vs 14°) for reverse shoulder arthroplasty in 40 patients in short-term, retrospective follow-up of 6 to 18 months.

SUMMARY

The physiologic age of the patient, fracture pattern, prospective head viability, and bone quality must all be taken into account to choose the correct treatment method for proximal humeral fractures. In young active patients, an anatomic reduction must be obtained for hope of a good outcome. Fractures with poor prognostic factors for head viability based on Hertel's radiographic criteria (metaphyseal extension <8 mm, medial hinge displacement >2 mm, or those with an anatomic neck component) are best treated with arthroplasty. The choice of hemiarthroplasty versus reverse total shoulder arthroplasty must be based on surgeon experience and patient expectations.

Fractures that are considered for fixation should be evaluated for bone quality by measuring combined cortical width. Most 2-part fractures may be treated with a sling, but for those with greater than 66% translation of a surgical neck fracture or tuberosity fracture with greater than 5 mm displacement, open reduction and internal fixation must be considered. Operative 2-part fractures with a combined cortical width of greater than 4 mm may be treated with CRPP, whereas those less than 4 mm combined cortical width should be treated with transosseous suture fixation. Three- and four-part fractures with greater than 4 mm combined cortical width and valgus impaction may be treated with open reduction internal fixation with a locked plate. Those with varus deformity or

less than 4 mm combined cortical width should have consideration for osteobiologic agent, bone graft or intramedullary strut graft for stable reduction, and ORIF with a locked plate.

REFERENCES

1. Lauritzen JB, Schwarz P, Lund B, et al. Changing incidence and residual lifetime risk of common osteoporosis-related fractures. Osteoporos Int 1993;3(3):127–32.
2. Hagino H, Fujiwara S, Nakashima E, et al. Case-control study of risk factors for fractures of the distal radius and proximal humerus among the Japanese population. Osteoporos Int 2004;15(3):226–30.
3. Palvanen M, Kannus P, Niemi S, et al. Update in the epidemiology of proximal humeral fractures. Clin Orthop Relat Res 2006;442:87–92.
4. Gerber C, Schneeberger AG, Vinh TS. The arterial vascularization of the humeral head. An anatomical study. J Bone Joint Surg Am 1990;72(10):1486–94.
5. Hettrich CM, Boraiah S, Dyke JP, et al. Quantitative assessment of the vascularity of the proximal part of the humerus. J Bone Joint Surg Am 2010;92(4):943–8.
6. Hertel R, Hempfing A, Stiehler M, et al. Predictors of humeral head ischemia after intracapsular fracture of the proximal humerus. J Shoulder Elbow Surg 2004;13(4):427–33.
7. Gallo RA, Sciulli R, Daffner RH, et al. Defining the relationship between rotator cuff injury and proximal humerus fractures. Clin Orthop Relat Res 2007;458:70–7.
8. Neer CS. Displaced proximal humeral fractures. I. Classification and evaluation. J Bone Joint Surg Am 1970;52(6):1077–89.
9. Marsh JL, Slongo TF, Agel J, et al. Fracture and dislocation classification compendium - 2007: Orthopaedic Trauma Association Classification, Database and Outcomes Committee. J Orthop Trauma 2007;21(Suppl 10):S1–133.
10. Tingart MJ, Apreleva M, Stechow von D, et al. The cortical thickness of the proximal humeral diaphysis predicts bone mineral density of the proximal humerus. J Bone Joint Surg Br 2003;85(4):611–7.
11. Gaebler C, McQueen MM, Court-Brown CM. Minimally displaced proximal humeral fractures: epidemiology and outcome in 507 cases. Acta Orthop Scand 2003;74(5):580–5.
12. Torrens C, Corrales M, Vilà G, et al. Functional and quality-of-life results of displaced and nondisplaced proximal humeral fractures treated conservatively. J Orthop Trauma 2011;25(10):581–7.
13. Yüksel HY, Yimaz S, Akşahin E, et al. The results of nonoperative treatment for three- and four-part fractures of the proximal humerus in low-demand patients. J Orthop Trauma 2011;25(10):588–95.

14. Panagopoulos AM, Dimakopoulos P, Tyllianakis M, et al. Valgus impacted proximal humeral fractures and their blood supply after transosseous suturing. Int Orthop 2004;28(6):333–7.

15. Rowles DJ, McGrory JE. Percutaneous pinning of the proximal part of the humerus. An anatomic study. J Bone Joint Surg Am 2001;83-A(11): 1695–9.

16. Gerber C, Werner CML, Vienne P. Internal fixation of complex fractures of the proximal humerus. J Bone Joint Surg Br 2004;86(6):848–55.

17. Olerud P, Ahrengart L, Ponzer S, et al. Internal fixation versus nonoperative treatment of displaced 3-part proximal humeral fractures in elderly patients: a randomized controlled trial. J Shoulder Elbow Surg 2011;20(5):747–55.

18. Fjalestad T, Hole MØ, Hovden IA, et al. Surgical treatment with an angular stable plate for complex displaced proximal humeral fractures in elderly patients: a randomized controlled trial. J Orthop Trauma 2012;26(2):98–106.

19. Sproul RC, Iyengar JJ, Devcic Z, et al. A systematic review of locking plate fixation of proximal humerus fractures. Injury 2011;42(4):408–13.

20. Zhu Y, Lu Y, Shen J, et al. Locking intramedullary nails and locking plates in the treatment of two-part proximal humeral surgical neck fractures: a prospective randomized trial with a minimum of three years of follow-up. J Bone Joint Surg Am 2011;93(2):159–68.

21. Neviaser AS, Hettrich CM, Beamer BS, et al. Endosteal strut augment reduces complications associated with proximal humeral locking plates. Clin Orthop Relat Res 2011;469(12):3300–6.

22. Kontakis G, Koutras C, Tosounidis T, et al. Early management of proximal humeral fractures with hemiarthroplasty: a systematic review. J Bone Joint Surg Br 2008;90(11):1407–13.

23. Gallinet D, Clappaz P, Garbuio P, et al. Three or four parts complex proximal humerus fractures: hemiarthroplasty versus reverse prosthesis: a comparative study of 40 cases. Orthop Traumatol Surg Res 2009; 95(1):48–55.

Emerging Concepts in Upper Extremity Trauma
Humeral Shaft Fractures

Robert J. Steffner, MD*, Mark A. Lee, MD

KEYWORDS

• Humeral shaft • Plate • Intramedullary nail • Radial nerve palsy • Nonunion

KEY POINTS

• Surgical indications for humeral shaft fractures are expanding.
• Elderly, osteoporotic humeral shaft fractures are becoming more common.
• Use of a plate or nail for fixation depends on fracture and patient characteristics as well as surgeon preference.
• Minimally invasive anterior plating has favorable outcomes.
• Most radial nerve palsies can be observed.
• Nonunion and bone defect management must consider the severity of initial injury, time since injury, patient comorbidities, and healing response to date.

INTRODUCTION

Fractures of the humeral shaft are common fractures in low-energy and high-energy trauma, and optimal clinical management remains controversial. Nonsurgical management has been supported as the preferred treatment based on high union rates and minimal functional deficit due to a rich vascular supply from overlying muscle and the wide motion available at the glenohumeral joint. Historically, surgical treatment, usually via plate fixation, has been less common outside of some very specific clinical situations, such as open fractures, ipsilateral forearm fractures, and fractures with concomitant vascular injuries. Recent studies of nonoperative management have challenged surgeons' understanding of these fractures and the perception of their favorable outcomes. Current considerations support expanded operative indications with traditional open-plate fixation as well as with the use of new minimally invasive techniques, new implants, and a reconsideration of intramedullary nailing.

EPIDEMIOLOGY

Humeral shaft fractures make up 3% to 5% of all fractures.[1] Distribution is bimodal with high-energy injuries occurring in young males and low-energy mechanisms taking place in elderly women. The latter is becoming more common.

CHARACTERISTICS AND DIAGNOSIS

Anatomically, the humeral shaft is the area between the proximal pectoralis major insertion and the distal metaphyseal flare. Fracture in this area presents with displacement and angulation that is representative of the energy involved and the pull of the muscular attachments above and below the fracture. On presentation, a history is initiated with emphasis on hand dominance, type

This work received institutional support only.
The authors have nothing to disclose.
Department of Orthopaedic Surgery, Ellison ACC, University of California-Davis, 4860 Y Street, Suite 1700, Sacramento, CA 95817, USA
* Corresponding author.
E-mail addresses: rsteffner@gmail.com; rjsteffner@ucdavis.edu

Orthop Clin N Am 44 (2013) 21–33
http://dx.doi.org/10.1016/j.ocl.2012.08.005

of work or hobby, and mechanism of injury. Low-energy mechanisms should heighten suspicion of pathologic fracture through tumor or metabolic disease. High-energy injuries should warrant higher suspicion for open fractures and compartment syndrome and further investigation for associated injuries to the lung, ribs, clavicle, scapula, brachial plexus, and axillary artery. A focused history should identify modifiable factors that influence healing, such as smoking and other medical comorbidities. Physical examination of the shoulder and upper extremity is paramount to assess the soft tissue injury and possible neurovascular sequelae. A detailed motor examination documenting active wrist extension must be verified as radial nerve palsy following fracture has an incidence of 6% to17%. Radial nerve injury is most common with transverse middiaphyseal fractures.[2] It is important not to accept digital extension as evidence of radial nerve function because hand intrinsics from the ulnar nerve can perform this function as well. In proximal shaft fractures, lateral shoulder skin sensation and the ability to push the elbow into the torso can be used to assess the axillary nerve. Standard orthogonal radiographs of the shoulder, humerus, and elbow should be obtained. With proximal or distal fractures, any suspicion of articular extension should be further evaluated with CT imaging. Initial management is aimed at pain control and immobilizing the fracture and can usually be achieved with a coaptation splint, sling and swath, or shoulder immobilizer. Acute functional bracing is becoming more common because it offers patients the immediate advantage of hygiene control and potential elbow motion once pain subsides.

MANAGEMENT

Most isolated humeral shaft fractures have been historically treated without surgery. In most patients, this fracture will heal predictably without surgical intervention because it is a well-vascularized bone encapsulated by muscle. Using a functional brace, Sarmiento and colleagues[3] reported a union rate of 97% in 620 subjects, including 94% union in low-grade open fractures. The high union rates coupled with the shoulder's ability to compensate for moderate degrees of deformity has traditionally made nonoperative treatment a reasonable first option in many patients. The limits of acceptable reduction are considered to be 20° of sagittal plane angulation, 30° of coronal angulation, 15° of malrotation, and 3 cm of shortening. These standards are historical, however, and the degree of disability was based on a sample of 32 subjects, only two of which had a malrotation deformity, and no objective

measures were used. Functional bracing maintains fracture alignment through gravity and soft tissue compression.

Enthusiasm for functional bracing has been challenged with recent observations of permanent loss of motion and a higher than expected nonunion rate of 10%.[4] Specific fracture patterns, most notably transverse and proximal-third oblique fractures may have unacceptably higher rates of nonunion.[4] Further, certain injury and patient factors make functional bracing less likely to succeed. These include plexus injury, in which muscle contractility around the fracture is lost and cannot provide the essential compression to maintain fracture alignment and prevent distraction, and morbid obesity, in which effective bracing technique is difficult and excess tissue often creates frontal plane malalignment.

Absolute indications continue to be open and pathologic fractures, associated vascular injuries requiring repair, brachial plexopathy, severe soft tissue injury precluding closed treatment, associated articular injury of the shoulder or elbow, and ipsilateral operative forearm fracture. Relative indications are guided by patient and fracture factors in addition to associated injuries. By discussing this with patients and understanding the demands of their lives, surgeons are able to make individual recommendations for conservative versus surgical management. Frequently, multiply injured patients with humeral shaft fractures and, occasionally, isolated shaft fractures in patients who need rapid return to function are treated surgically. Surgical management can allow immediate full range of motion, pain control, early rehabilitation, and return to work. However, risks of radial nerve palsy, reoperation, infection, anesthetic risk, bleeding, and nonunion must be discussed and accepted by the patient before proceeding.

EXTERNAL FIXATION

Use of external fixation is generally limited to damage control situations in which patients are unable to physiologically tolerate extensive surgical intervention. Additional indications include associated soft tissue injury requiring multiple debridements or frequent dressing changes, vascular injuries requiring bony stabilization before repair, and joint instability. Risks with external fixation include pin loosening, infection, lost motion, refracture, malunion, and nonunion. The radial nerve is also at risk during distal percutaneous pin insertion. A recent study of 40 cadaver upper extremities, demonstrated four radial nerve injuries and nine pins with direct contact with the nerve during percutaneous pin insertion. The investigators ecommended larger incisions with blunt dissection to the lateral humeral cortex, finger palpation or the nerve, and retraction of tissues during pin nsertion to avoid injury.[5]

In damage control situations, once the patient is hemodynamically stable, consideration must be given to definitive management. This often requires conversion to an internal fixation construct and associated debridement and wound coverage in njuries with soft tissue compromise. A retrospective study was done of 17 humeral shaft fractures nitially treated with damage-control external fixators that were converted to plates at an average of 6.2 days; 14 days was the longest duration. Eighty-eight percent healed. Two subjects developed infections requiring debridement and conversion back to external fixation. Their failure was attributed to poor compliance and severity of initial njury. Conversion to plate was thought to be safe within 2 weeks.[6] There are no data to suggest a safe time point for conversion to an intramedullary nail.

INTRAMEDULLARY NAILING

Intramedullary nailing of long-bone fractures has been very effective in the lower extremities but historically limited in the upper extremity owing to concerns of shoulder and elbow dysfunction,

nonunion, and reoperation. Further, there is long-standing concern regarding stiffness from capsular adhesion, pain, and fracture at joints adjacent to start sites on antegrade and retrograde nails. The theoretical benefits are significant and include smaller incisions, maintenance of fracture hematoma, and an implant that is load-sharing and can be used to ad lib immediately. Indications for intramedullary fixation have been narrower than plate fixation and include fractures with associated soft tissue injury precluding an open approach, pathologic fractures, extreme osteopenia, and true diaphyseal segmental patterns.

Recent advances in technique, implants, surgeon experience, and improved study design have renewed interest in intramedullary nailing. The anterolateral acromial approach using the interval between the anterior and middle deltoid raphe leads to better visualization of the rotator cuff, making it easier to identify the rotator interval itself and pinpoint the start site. Moreover, the start site with this approach is more collinear with the intramedullary canal, making it technically easier to avoid varus malalignment and to achieve medial calcar contact (**Fig. 1**). It also allows for protection of the anterior branch of the axillary nerve during placement of proximal interlocking bolts. With respect to the start site on the humerus, translation of the entry site medially onto the articular surface

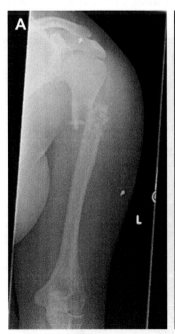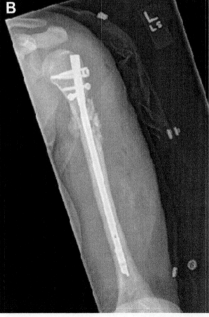

Fig. 1. Comminuted proximal humeral shaft fracture. (*A*) Deltoid pull on the distal fragment leads to displacement and a high rate of nonunion in this fracture pattern. Relative stability with an intramedullary nail spans the comminution without disrupting the biology. (*B*) A well-placed entry site avoids medial displacement of the distal fragment and varus malalignment.

will avoid the common deformity of medial shaft displacement with nail passage.

Nails today are larger, more rigid, anatomically-contoured, and statically locked with multiple proximal and distal interlocks. They share load with the bone and avoid stress shielding. Use of newer nails with minimal reaming has been shown to reduce nonunion and implant failure.[7] Patients with native isthmus diameters of 9 mm or greater are good candidates for nails because they can accommodate a larger nail with minimal reaming. New designs with more points of fixation have expanded the level of proximal and distal fractures that can be nailed. There is increasing interest in straight proximal nails with a more articular, on-axis start site. These are optimal for proximal fractures and assist in avoidance of frontal plane malalignment. Many of these nails have multiple proximal locking options and the ability to achieve angular stability with the interlocking screws (**Fig. 2**). As a result, use of intramedullary nails have increased and, as surgeons have become more comfortable with the technique and radiographic interpretations during the surgery, common complications, such as subacromial impingement due to prominent nails, rotator cuff tears due to poor technique during canal access, and serial reaming, have become less common.

Many technical tricks during intramedullary nailing can be used to avoid complications. One such priority is protection of the radial nerve. Pushing the reamer across the fracture site protects the radial nerve from the reamer itself and from thermal injury. Isolating the nerve through a small, separate incision and directly visualizing it during canal reaming is also possible and reassuring (**Fig. 3**). To avoid a prominent proximal nail tip and achieve fracture site compression, countersinking the nail by 3 to 4 mm and backslapping to cortical contact or using new nail designs that allow for interfragmentary compression after distal interlocking has decreased the number of nonunions.[1] For proximal humeral shaft fractures undergoing antegrade nailing, restoration of the medial column prevents loss of reduction, screw penetration into the glenohumeral joint, and lost humeral head height. This reduction can be attained by tagging the rotator cuff tendons and placing two 2 mm Kirschner wires into the humeral head and using these as joysticks to control sagittal and coronal alignment. A Kirschner wire, outside of the expected path of the nail, can then be placed across the fracture for provisional stabilization. A recent review of 48 subjects treated with a contemporary antegrade humeral nail demonstrated 96% union in a mean time of 10 weeks, five required reoperation for nonunion, loose hardware, and infection. Ninety-one percent had excellent or good shoulder function.[8] In another study, 94% of subjects went onto uncomplicated union with good functional outcomes. This study highlighted that most complications are the result of surgeon technical error and not limitations of the nailing technique. In addition,

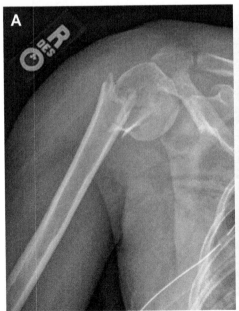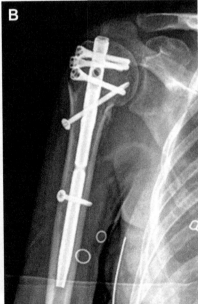

Fig. 2. (*A*) Comminuted surgical neck fracture in a polytrauma patient. Reduction and fixation with a new intramedullary nail with multiple proximal locking options for angular stability. (*B*) The straight proximal geometry of the nail and articular on-axis start site avoids frontal plane malalignment.

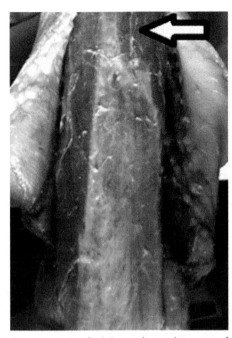

Fig. 3. Approximately 2.5 cm above the apex of the triceps aponeurosis, the radial nerve (*arrow*) lies in the spiral groove. This reliable landmark can be used to identify the radial nerve through a limited incision.

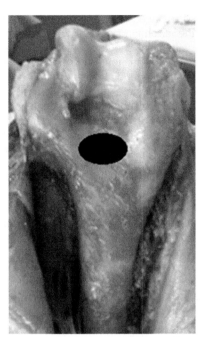

Fig. 4. Entry site for retrograde humeral nailing. Roof of the olecranon fossa creates a path that is more in line with the intramedullary canal, reducing the chance of iatrogenic supracondylar fracture.

the investigators noted that younger subjects had better shoulder outcomes than elderly subjects did. Despite the worse outcomes, elderly subjects tolerated their deficits well because of their lower functional requirements.[9] Healing and acceptable functional results seem possible with precise technique. Improved recognition of technical issues, such as placement of the entry site, fracture site compression, and understanding newer implant options, is imperative for treatment success.

Antegrade nailing is favored in North America, but there is persistent regional interest in locked retrograde nailing technique. Retrograde nails can be used for fractures in the distal-third and middle-third of the humerus in patients with shoulder abduction greater than 60°. A new technique with the patient supine, using a radiolucent arm table and the elbow fully flexed, splits the triceps tendon and establishes the nail entry point between the supracondylar ridges through the superior aspect of the olecranon fossa (**Fig. 4**). This entry site provides straighter access to the canal and remains clear of the olecranon tip of the ulna during full elbow extension. The proximal insertion of the nail is generally to about 1.5 cm below the humeral head articular surface. A large enough entry site is crucial in retrograde nailing because unforceful introduction of the nail avoids iatrogenic supracondylar fractures. Reaming is

not necessary as long as a rigid nail can be passed. However, it is recommended to ream 2 mm larger than the nail at the insertion and 1.5 mm larger in the isthmus and proximal humerus to avoid supracondylar fracture. A study of 16 subjects using this technique reported no iatrogenic fractures.[10] Although useful in preventing bending moments and nail incarceration, canal reaming weakens the humerus and does not prevent deformity from off axis entry sites. The bony anatomy of the distal humerus makes it necessary to remove more bone to accommodate current nail designs. Avoidance of the creation of a scenario of bone loss and supracondylar humerus fracture in a poorly performed retrograde nail is critical.

Antegrade nailing is more forgiving because less bone must be removed to accommodate current nail designs. There is growing interest in the use of straight nails for proximal-third and proximal shaft fractures. Most commonly done supine with a medial scapular bump on a reversed table with a radiolucent foot extension or in the beach chair position, a 2 to 3 cm incision is made from the anterolateral tip of the acromion heading toward the deltoid tuberosity. The fibers of the anterior and middle heads of the deltoid are bluntly divided. The start site is identified with a guide pin, which should be aiming to the center of the intramedullary canal on the anteroposterior and lateral fluoroscopic projections. This site is typically anterior to the acromion but can be more easily accessed with slight shoulder extension. The guide pin should translate toward the articular surface on the anteroposterior to avoid varus deformity. In addition, this more medial start site protects the less vascular and more distal tendinous footprint of the supraspinatus. Once identified, care is taken to adequately visualize and split the rotator cuff tendons and tag them with suture to safely mobilize the ends out of the way of the opening reamer. The importance of diligence during this step cannot be overemphasized. It is easier to mobilize the tendons with a more medial start site. Antegrade intramedullary nailing is technically easier to perform and has become the predominant technique in humeral nailing.

Part of the renewed interest in intramedullary nailing has been brought on by the demographic changes highlighted earlier. A greater proportion of humeral shaft fractures presenting through emergency departments are elderly individuals with low-energy falls and poor bone quality. The use of a load sharing implant is very appealing to treat these patients. Fast stabilization with early rehabilitation to allow return home and continued independence is the priority in treating these individuals.

PLATE FIXATION

Long considered the preferred mode of treatment because of reliable union, lower reoperation, and less effect on adjacent joints, internal fixation has the drawbacks of direct fracture exposure, blood loss, and potential iatrogenic radial nerve palsy. One of the distinct advantages of plating is the ability to tailor the plating construct to the personality of the fracture. Simple fractures receive compression plating (**Fig. 5**). Comminuted segments undergo bridge plating techniques (**Fig. 6**). Fractures with poor bone quality can be augmented with locking or hybrid constructs. Long plates with greater working length are used to create relative stability constructs in comminuted fractures that allow micromotion to promote healing. Dynamic compression plates of 4.5 mm can accommodate patient anatomy and provide stout plates that can tolerate early weight-bearing.[11] They are designed with staggered holes to improve screw density and prevent fracture propagation. Fractures in proximity to joints can be plated with periarticular precontoured plates that match the proximal or distal anatomy of the humerus, effectively reducing the amount of operative anesthetic because surgeons no longer have to mold plates to fit anatomic contours. Humeral shaft fractures with bone loss can be shortened up to 2 cm without affecting muscle strength and improves healing by allowing cortical apposition and compression.

Surgical approach has traditionally been dictated by the location of the fracture with proximal and middle shaft fractures using an anterolateral approach and distal-third shaft fractures a posterior approach, either triceps-splitting or triceps-sparing. In an effort to reduce the frequency of iatrogenic radial nerve palsies, a straight anterior approach has come into vogue with its application most commonly seen with minimally invasive plating.

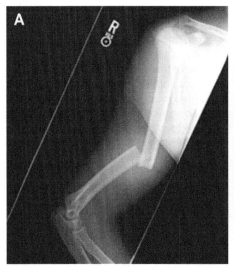
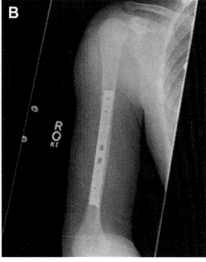

Fig. 5. (*A*) Transverse middiaphyseal fracture of the humeral shaft is at higher risk of nonunion with conservative management due to distraction forces and gapping across the fracture. (*B*) Postoperative radiograph after a posterior approach and compression plating.

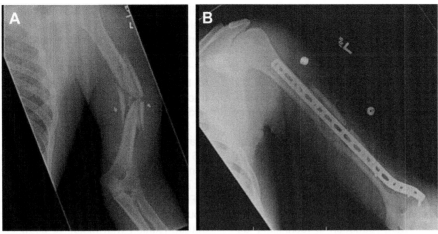

Fig. 6. (*A*) Closed comminuted middiaphyseal humeral shaft fracture with a primary radial nerve palsy. (*B*) Posterior bridge plate using a posterolateral periarticular distal humerus plate. The radial nerve was explored mainly to assure the plate slid underneath.

Minimally invasive plating osteosynthesis (MIPO) can be performed on the humerus with submuscular anteromedial and anterolateral plating. It is indicated in shaft fractures at least 6 cm below the surgical neck and 6 cm above the coronoid fossa to accommodate six cortices of fixation on each side. The patient is positioned supine on a radiolucent table with the arm in 90° of abduction in full supination. The surgeon stands cephalad to the arm and the C-arm comes from the axilla. A 4 cm incision is made 5 cm distal to the anterior acromion and along the deltoid tuberosity. The interval between the bicep tendon and the deltoid insertion is developed. A second 4 cm incision is made 5 cm proximal to the elbow flexion crease in-line with the lateral bicep tendon. The brachialis muscle is split in its middle-third and lateral-third junction. This goes between the musculocutaneous and radial nerves. A narrow 10-hole or 12-hole, straight, 4.5 mm plate is tunneled submuscular along the straight corridor of bone in this location. The fracture is then reduced, usually with closed manipulation (**Fig. 7**).[12] Advantages of this technique are more cosmetic incisions, less soft tissue

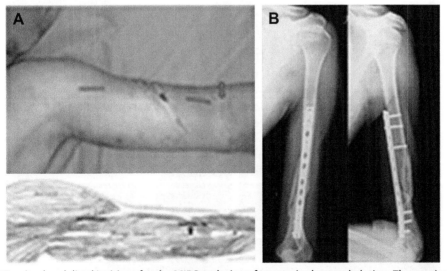

Fig. 7. (*A*) Proximal and distal incisions for the MIPO technique for anterior humeral plating. The proximal incision uses the interval between the bicep and deltoid. The distal incision goes lateral to the bicep and splits the brachialis. The forearm is supinated. The red arrow notes the elbow flexion crease. (*B*) A distal-third humeral shaft fracture 3 months after being treated with anterior MIPO plating. The radiographs demonstrate a favorable healing response. (*From* Zhiquan A, Bingfang Z, Yeming W, et al. Minimally invasive plating osteosynthesis (MIPO) of middle and distal-third humeral shaft fractures. J Orthop Trauma 2007;21:628–33; with permission from JOT.)

dissection, preserved biologic environment at the fracture, use of a true internervous plane, and protection of the radial nerve. MIPO is particularly safe in the presence of a radial nerve palsy because recovery is unaffected by the procedure. Criticisms of this approach include putting the plate on the compression side of the fracture, the difficulty obtaining an adequate reduction, lost elbow range of motion postoperatively, and risk to the radial and musculocutaneous nerve with percutaneous screw placement. Plating the compression side of the fracture is theoretically a disadvantage. Healing time, however, is equivalent to plating the tension or posterior side. Tension side plating is thought to be of less consequence in a non–weight-bearing long bone. Fracture reduction is technically demanding in MIPO and requires experience. Techniques to avoid malreduction include abducting the arm to avoid varus malalignment and flexing the elbow 30° with longitudinal traction to avoid sagittal plane deformity. Early motion can prevent brachial scarring and loss of elbow motion and must be instituted. Percutaneous screw placement places several nerves at risk. A study of 18 cadaveric arms with 10-hole limited contact plates placed via MIPO showed the radial nerve is at risk in the midportion of the arm with bicortical screws and that the musculocutaneous nerve crosses anterior

to the plate, 13.5 cm distal to the greater tuberosity Apivatthakakul and colleagues[13] recommend unicortical screws in the midportion of the arm and extending incisions for direct visualization to place additional screws. This technique can also be used to bridge comminuted and segmental humerus fractures. Ninety percent union with good elbow and shoulder functional outcomes was reported on 21 subjects treated with AO Type C humeral shaft fractures treated with MIPO and combination 4.5 mm plates. Initial cortical screws are used for compression and then followed by locking screws for added torsional stability.[12]

Fractures of the distal-third shaft continue to be troublesome. Too short for nailing, getting adequate fixation with plates to allow early motion has been challenging (**Fig. 8**). A recent surgical technique using dual plating through a single posterior midline incision has shown good results with respect to union and maintaining alignment while allowing early motion. This technique uses 90-90 plating with a lateral 2.7 or 3.5 mm pelvic reconstruction plate with or without a lag screw to reduce and stabilize the fracture. A precontoured 3.5 mm combination posterolateral plate used in compression, locking, or bridging based on patient and fracture characteristics, is then placed to achieve rigid stabilization (**Fig. 9**).[14]

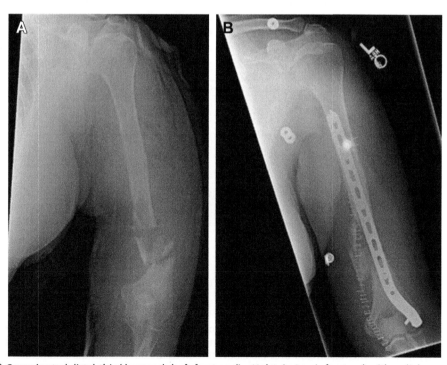

Fig. 8. (A) Comminuted distal-third humeral shaft fracture (ie, Holstein-Lewis fracture) with radial nerve palsy. (B) Open reduction and internal fixation with nerve exploration performed with use of a long distal humerus posterolateral periarticular plate.

A **B**

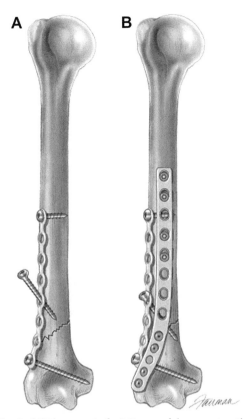

Fig. 9. (*A*) Placement of a 3.5 mm pelvic reconstruction plate, straight lateral with placement of a lag screw, using the plate as a washer. (*B*) A posterolateral precontoured 3.5 mm plate is then added to neutralize the construct. (*From* Prasarn ML, Ahn J, Paul O, et al. Dual plating for fractures of the distal-third of the humeral shaft. J Orthop Trauma 2011;25:57–63; with permission from JOT.)

RECENT REVIEWS OF PLATING VERSUS INTRAMEDULLARY NAILING

Studies with modern nails and experienced surgeons have recently demonstrated locked nails to be equivalent in union and functional outcomes compared with compression plates for humeral shaft fractures. A meta-analysis establishing higher shoulder impingement and reoperation with humeral nailing was recently updated and showed no statistical difference in total complications, nonunion, infection, nerve palsy, or reoperation between plates and nails. A retrospective review of 91 subjects demonstrated no difference in fracture union and reoperation. Plating had more iatrogenic radial nerve palsies, whereas intramedullary nailing had more iatrogenic fractures and elbow symptoms with retrograde nails and shoulder symptoms with antegrade nails.[15] Malrotation is a concern with diaphyseal humerus fractures along with length

and alignment. It is suspected that malrotation in internal rotation greater than 20° increases contact between the humeral head and the glenoid. This may lead to advanced shoulder degeneration.

OPEN FRACTURES

Open fractures are higher-energy injuries with varying degrees of soft tissue disruption. Low-grade open fractures can be treated with an emergency department washout, antibiotics, and functional bracing, and, although the well-vascularized brachium makes this possible, this treatment option is reserved for poor surgical candidates. High-grade open fractures produce soft tissue insults that require aggressive operative debridement and stabilization. Immediate plating of open fractures is safe for most open humerus fractures. In a recent study, 46 subjects with open fractures ranging from Gustilo and Anderson grade I to IIIC, received debridement, irrigation, intravenous antibiotics, and open reduction and internal fixation in the same sitting. Eight-seven percent healed without complication. There were six delayed unions, no deep infections, and no reoperation for nonunion. The investigators concluded that immediate plate fixation in conjunction with thorough open fracture management was the treatment of choice.[16] Any grade open fracture associated with radial nerve palsy remains an indication for operative debridement, nerve exploration, and surgical stabilization of the fracture.

PATHOLOGIC FRACTURES

Suspicion of a primary malignancy should warrant referral to an orthopedic oncologist. Most instances of pathologic lesions in the humerus are overwhelmingly the sequelae of known metastatic disease. Bone is the third most common site of metastatic lesions and the humerus is commonly involved. These fractures occur late in the disease process and with low-energy mechanisms. Thirty-five percent of individuals live greater than 1 year after pathologic fracture. With this increase in life expectancy, pain control, restoring function, and improving quality of life become the priorities in addressing these fractures. Intramedullary nailing is an effective means of stabilization because it protects a long segment, can be performed quickly, and has small incisions allowing earlier adjunct radiotherapy. Cement augmentation of humeral nails may provide better pain relief and immediate return of function. The cement may provide greater rigidity and decrease local tumor mass without inhibiting healing. This technique, however, is technically challenging. Impending fracture can also be an indication for intramedullary stabilization of the humerus. General indications for prophylactic fixation are diaphyseal lytic lesions and lesions with 75% or greater cortical loss.

BONE DEFECTS

High-energy open injuries or high-velocity gunshot wounds are often accompanied by soft tissue and bone defects. In these instances, an induced membrane technique is frequently used. After adequate debridement that may require temporary external fixation or bridge plating, conversion to an intramedullary nail or repeat bridge plating with maintenance of the defect site with a cement block spacer and soft tissue coverage is performed. Six weeks or more later, when the soft tissue coverage is mature, the cement block is removed and replaced with bone graft. The graft is contained and supported by the biologic membrane formed around the cement spacer. The authors' preference for graft material includes autograft from the iliac crest or marrow reaming obtained from the femur with a Reamer-Irrigator-Aspirator (Synthes USA, West Chester, PA, USA) combined with bone marrow aspirate and extended in cases requiring more graft volume with allograft cancellous bone and demineralized bone matrix, which has potential inductive function and improves graft handling in large defects; it can be as effective as iliac crest bone graft in the treatment of humeral

shaft nonunions. Alternatively, at the time of conversion to an intramedullary nail, a spine cage can be filled with graft and placed into the defect. The nail is then passed through the cage and locked into place (**Fig. 10**).

OSTEOPOROSIS

Humeral shaft fractures are becoming more common in the elderly.[1] Fixation is challenging and surgical failure can be catastrophic as nonunion is poorly tolerated in the elderly. These patients are less able to adapt and effectively use their contralateral upper extremity. Intramedullary nails have the advantage of being load-sharing devices that maintain the soft tissue envelope around the fracture. Nails provide relative stability to fractures that are frequently comminuted. Locking plate technology is an alternative. This construct is linked and performs as one unit. To fail, all screws must loosen, as opposed to compression plating in which individual screws can fail. If a plate is chosen to treat an osteoporotic fracture, posterior plating with a narrow 4.5 mm combination plate is often adequate. Two locking screws on each side of the fracture zone are the minimum requirement. Two screws in each fracture fragment provide equivalent axial, bending, and torsional strength compared with three screws. Load to failure in torsion is higher with two screws compared with three. Torsional stiffness is greater with plates than with nails.

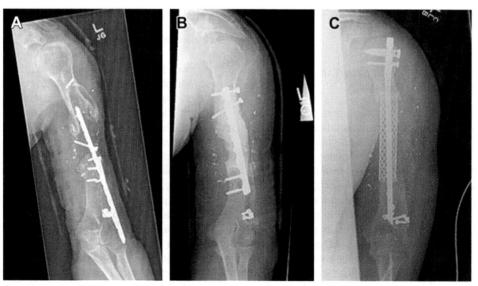

Fig. 10. (*A*) Long-standing humeral shaft segmental bone loss from an initial high-energy gunshot wound with multiple failed attempts at fixation. (*B*) Stage one of reconstruction included debridement, culture, antibiotic spacer with temporary stabilization. (*C*) After 6 weeks of intravenous antibiotics and an appropriate antibiotic holiday, the patient was reconstructed with a titanium mesh spine cage filled with bone graft to rebuild bone stock, all supported with an intramedullary nail.

Plating constructs can be augmented with onlay cortical allograft or segmental fibular allograft placed on the cortex opposite the plate and captured with the plate screws (**Fig. 11**). Fibular allograft can also be placed intramedullary through existing fracture lines and used to facilitate reduction through pushing screws. This construct improves fixation strength and ultimate stability during early rehabilitation.

RADIAL NERVE PALSY

Radial nerve palsy complicates 11.8% of humeral shaft fractures. Palsies occurring at the time of injury in closed fractures recover 90% of the time in an average of 7 weeks.[17] Radial nerve palsy in conjunction with open fracture and penetrating injury has a greater chance of direct insult to the nerve and a lower spontaneous recovery rate.[17] Early exploration is recommended. This allows assessment of the nerve for direct damage and avoids later dissection through scar and callus. Primary repair does poorly; however, early knowledge of direct nerve injury can guide patient prognostic discussions and preparation for reconstructive nerve grafting or tendon transfer procedures. Long oblique middle-third to distal-third shaft fractures, known as Holstein-Lewis fractures, have a higher incidence of radial nerve palsy in closed fractures. The recovery is equivalent to other palsies in closed humeral shaft fractures and warrants nonoperative management.

A recent paper demonstrated that outcome of radial nerve function is influenced by the initial trauma. High-energy injuries, defined as motor vehicle collisions, falls from height, and crush mechanisms, had a low recovery rate. Those that improved took almost twice as long to return than low-energy palsies did. The investigators recommended expectantly following high-energy palsies for at least 6 months after recovery and informing these patients early about their poor prognosis and possible need for tendon transfers after bone and soft tissue healing. Bishop and Ring[18] did an expected-value analysis of the management of radial nerve palsies and acknowledged the difficulty in making this decision under conditions of uncertainty. They concluded that observation is the optimal management strategy and that a 40% or less estimation of recovery is necessary to indicate operative exploration.

Nonunion

Nonunion is the failure to heal and may be due to patient factors, fracture characteristics, or a combination of the two. Patient factors include poor nutrition, medical comorbidities, alcohol use, and poor compliance. Fracture factors include open fractures, midshaft transverse or short oblique

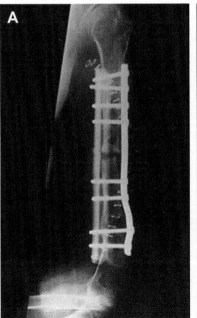
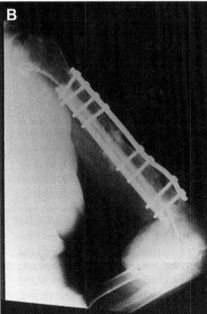

Fig. 11. (*A*) Aseptic nonunion of the humeral shaft treated with anterior femoral shaft allograft cortical onlay with posterior compression plating. (*B*) Radiograph union evident at 3-months postoperatively. (*From* Hornicek FJ, Zych GA, Hutson JJ, et al. Salvage of humeral nonunions with onlay bone plate allograft augmentation. Clin Orthop Relat Res 2001;386:203–9; with permission from CORR.)

patterns, comminution, unstable fixation, and fracture gapping. Patients typically present with pain but can complain of persistent fracture site movement. No precise timeline exists for defining a nonunion. The general guideline is 3 months for a delayed union and 6 months to declare a nonunion. Infection should always be assessed as a cause of nonunion in postoperative patients. Laboratory markers should be drawn preoperatively and multiple cultures taken at the time of operative debridement. Confirmed infection typically leads to staged management with implant removal, debridement, bone recanalization, antibiotic cement spacer, temporary stabilization, and intravenous antibiotics specific to the cultured organism. Once the infection is eradicated, the nonunion can be addressed in the same manner as an aseptic nonunion.

The first step in management of an aseptic nonunion is correct characterization between hypertrophic and atrophic causes because their treatments are distinct. Once established as a hypertrophic nonunion, treatment is straightforward and frequently only requires aggressive compression across interposed fibrous tissue with expected transformation to bone. Intramedullary fixation is a consideration in these nonunions because compression can be achieved with new nail designs and with less surgical soft tissue insult. Established nonunions may form a pseudarthrosis and this can be very challenging because it typically requires extensive debridement and resection of scar and pseudocapsule with subsequent compression plating. Most of these debridements are extensive and the authors uniformly perform autogenous bone grafting despite the cause. Atrophic nonunions frequently occur in high-energy and open fractures and require both biologic and mechanical stability. Autogenous iliac crest bone graft is an excellent source of cells and growth factors and is effective in treating nonunions.[19] It is not, however, without consequence because significant donor site morbidity occurs with harvest of the cells. Favorable results with autologous bone marrow concentrate with demineralized bone matrix suggest this may be a reasonable alternative for biologic stability. In treating an atrophic nonunion, any previous hardware should be removed, the pseudarthrosis or nonviable tissue around the bone ends should be resected, cortical shingling or scoring of the periosteum on both sides of the nonunion is done, followed by implant placement, which is most commonly a large fragment straight plate. The plate is then applied in compression with or without hybrid fixation depending on bone quality. These nonunions are uniformly grafted. This construct has demonstrated excellent rates of healing with few complications. Long bone cortical onlay allograft or segmental fibular allograft can be used to augment structural support in nonunions. Fixation is obtained through the plate screws opposite the graft. The allograft may provide some osteoinductive factors and incorporates well into native cortical bone by 3 months (see **Fig. 11**).

Proximal-third fractures make up 25% of all humeral shaft fractures, yet make up 53% of all nonunions.[20] Commonly, these fractures are initially treated with functional bracing and do not heal owing to the deforming forces of the deltoid. These can be treated with dual lateral and anterolateral compression plating and bone grafting.

Nonunion after intramedullary nailing is most often treated with nail removal and compression plating. Exchange nailing is not indicated and dynamization is not an option because the upper extremity receives distractive forces with upright posture. New nail designs, however, may allow treatment of delayed unions and nonunions with a small surgery through the original nail. Aparo and colleagues[21] looked at seven nonunions in subjects treated with retrograde unreamed humeral nails. Up to 20 months after injury, they were able to perform isolated interfragmentary compression through the nail. They achieved union in all subjects. Their study is underpowered but suggests that this may be an option in younger individuals with good bone stock.

In elderly patients unable to tolerate surgery or in patients unwilling to consider harvest of autogenous bone graft or the prospect of cadaveric graft Teriparatide (Forteo, Eli Lilly, Indianapolis, IN, USA) may be an alternative. Teriparatide is the first 34 amino acids of parathyroid hormone. It works by stimulating osteoblasts and, therefore, enhances ossification of endochondral callus. It works particularly well in trabecular bone but also enhances healing in cortical bone. In a recent case report, a 6-month-old humeral shaft nonunion after retrograde elastic nailing achieved union after 5 months of daily subcutaneous injections of Teriparatide.[22]

REHABILITATION

Multiple long bone fractures create mobilization issues, especially with lower extremity fractures in conjunction with humeral shaft fractures. Fixation with a 4.5 mm dynamic compression plate or a rigid, statically locked intramedullary nail will allow early weight-bearing for mobilization with crutches or a walker.[11] Early active motion of the shoulder and elbow is paramount. Posterior approaches should limit resisted extension for 4 to 6 weeks to protect the triceps.

SUMMARY

Fractures of the humeral shaft have expanding surgical indications because functional outcomes with conservative management are more fully appreciated. New nail designs may expand the use of intramedullary devices, especially in proximal fractures. Use of plating versus nailing depends on fracture and patient characteristics, as well as surgeon preference. Minimally invasive anterior plating has shown favorable outcomes and merits further study. Elderly shaft fractures are increasingly common and are best treated with hybrid plating or intramedullary nailing. Pathologic and impeding fractures are still best treated with intramedullary nails. Most radial nerve palsies, outside of those associated with high-grade open fractures, are best observed. Nonunion and bone defect management are challenging and may require multiple treatment modalities. Outcomes may be related to the severity of the initial injury.

REFERENCES

1. McKee MD. Fractures of the shaft of the humerus. In: Bucholz RW, Heckman JD, Court-Brown C, editors. Rockwood and Green's: fractures in adults. 6th edition. Philadelpha: Lippincott Williams & Wilkins; 2006. p. 1117–59.
2. Templeman DC, Sems SA. Humeral shaft fractures. In: Stannard JP, Schmidt AH, Kregor PJ, editors. Surgical treatment of orthopaedic trauma. 1st edition. New York: Thieme; 2007. p. 263–84.
3. Sarmiento A, Zagorski J, Zych G, et al. Functional bracing for the treatment of fractures of the humeral diaphysis. J Bone Joint Surg Am 2000;82:478–86.
4. Rutgers M, Ring D. Treatment of diaphyseal fractures of the humerus using a functional brace. J Orthop Trauma 2006;20:597–601.
5. Clement H, Pichler W, Tesch NP, et al. Anatomical basis of the risk of radial nerve injury related to the technique of external fixation applied to the distal humerus. Surg Radiol Anat 2010;32:221–4.
6. Suzuki T, Hak DJ, Stahel PF, et al. Safety and efficacy of conversion from external fixation to plate fixation in humeral shaft fractures. J Orthop Trauma 2010;24:414–9.
7. Riemer BL, Foglesong ME, Burke CJ 3rd, et al. Complications of Seidel intramedullary nailing of narrow diameter humeral diaphyseal fractures. Orthopedics 1994;17:19–29.
8. Tsourvakas S, Alexandropoulos C, Papachristos I, et al. Treatment of humeral shaft fractures with antegrade intramedullary locking nail. Musculoskelet Surg 2011;95:193–8.
9. Iacobellis C, Agro T, Aldegheri R. Locked antegrade intramedullary nailing of humeral shaft fractures. Musculoskelet Surg 2012;96:342–52.
10. Hollister AM, Saulsbery C, Odom JL, et al. New technique for humeral shaft fracture retrograde intramedullary nailing. Tech Hand Up Extrem Surg 2011; 15:138–43.
11. Patel R, Neu CP, Curtiss S, et al. Crutch weightbearing on comminuted humeral shaft fractures: a biomechanical comparison of large versus small fragment fixation for humeral shaft fractures. J Orthop Trauma 2011;5:300–5.
12. Jiang R, Luo CF, Zeng BF, et al. Minimally invasive plating for complex humeral shaft fractures. Arch Orthop Trauma Surg 2007;127:531–5.
13. Apivatthakakul T, Patiyasikan S, Luevitoonvechkit S. Danger zone for locking screw placement in minimally invasive plate osteosynthesis (MIPO) of humeral shaft fractures: a cadaveric study. Injury 2010;41:169–72.
14. Prasarn ML, Ahn J, Paul O, et al. Dual plating for fractures of the distal third of the humeral shaft. J Orthop Trauma 2011;25:57–63.
15. Denes E, Nus S, Sermon A, et al. Operative treatment of humeral shaft fractures. comparison of plating and intramedullary nailing. Acta Orthop Belg 2010;76:735–42.
16. Connolly S, McKee MD, Zdero R, et al. Immediate plate osteosynthesis of open fractures of the humeral shaft. J Trauma 2010;69:685–90.
17. Pollock FH, Drake D, Bovill EG, et al. Treatment of radial neuropathy associated with fractures of the humerus. J Bone Joint Surg Am 1981;63:239–43.
18. Bishop J, Ring D. Management of radial nerve palsy associated with humeral shaft fracture: a decision analysis model. J Hand Surg 2009;34A:991–6.
19. Lin CL, Fang CK, Chiu FY, et al. Revision with dynamic compression plate and cancellous bone graft for aseptic nonunion after surgical treatment of humeral shaft fracture. J Trauma 2009;67:1393–6.
20. Tytherleigh-Strong G, Walls N, McQueen MM. The epidemiology of humeral shaft fractures. J Bone Joint Surg Br 1998;80:249–53.
21. Apard T, Ducellier F, Hubert L, et al. Isolated interfragmentary compression for nonunion of humeral shaft fractures initially treated by nailing: a preliminary report of seven cases. Injury 2010;41:1262–5.
22. Oleo-Alvaro A, Moreno E. Atrophic humeral shaft nonunion treated with teriparatide (rh PTH 1-34). J Shoulder Elbow Surg 2010;19:e22–8.

Intra-Articular Distal Humerus Fractures

Anna N. Miller, MD[a], Daphne M. Beingessner, MD[b],*

KEYWORDS

- Distal humerus • Fracture • Articular injury elbow • Fixation • Elbow arthroplasty • Intra-articular

KEY POINTS

- Distal humerus fractures are relatively uncommon orthopedic injuries, representing less than 7% of adult fractures, and approximately 30% of fractures about the elbow.
- Most intra-articular distal humerus fractures require operative fixation for an anatomic reduction and to allow for early motion to optimize outcome.
- There are multiple approaches to the elbow joint including triceps-sparing, triceps-splitting, triceps-reflecting, and olecranon osteotoy.
- Total elbow arthroplasty is an option for management of these fractures in elderly osteoporotic patients.

Distal humerus fractures are relatively uncommon orthopedic injuries, representing less than 7% of adult fractures, and approximately 30% of fractures about the elbow.[1] Lateral column injuries are more common than medial column injuries, and multiple types have been described. In addition, distal humerus fractures commonly occur in two population groups: young people with a high energy mechanism and elderly people due to a low energy mechanism such as a fall, usually in association with osteoporosis. The incidence of these fractures may be increasing, especially as the population continues to age.

ANATOMY

Bony Anatomy

The elbow joint is composed of three bones (radius, ulna, and humerus) and comprises the ulnohumeral, radiocapitellar, and proximal radioulnar joints. The ulnohumeral joint is a hinge that allows for flexion and extension of the elbow. The axis of rotation of this joint is in slight external rotation (3°–9°) and valgus (4°–8°) from the humeral shaft.[1] The semilunar notch of the ulna engages with the trochlea and this close articulation gives bony stability. The trochlea itself is contained between the lateral and medial columns of the elbow, and it is covered with articular cartilage over 300° of its surface.[2] The medial and lateral columns diverge from the humeral shaft: the lateral column at approximately 20° and the medial column at approximately 45°. The distal articular surface is also angulated anterior to the shaft of the humerus, with approximately 30° to 40° anterior angulation of the capitellum and 25° anterior angulation of the trochlea.[2]

Ligamentous Anatomy and Articular Surface

The medial epicondyle is the distal extent of the medial column. The medial collateral ligament and flexor/pronator musculature originate from this area of the distal humerus. Similarly, on the lateral column, the lateral collateral ligament and extensor musculature originate on the lateral epicondyle. On

The authors have nothing to disclose, and no funding was received for this work.

a Department of Orthopaedic Surgery, Wake Forest University School of Medicine, Medical Center Boulevard, Winston-Salem, NC 27157-1070, USA; b Department of Orthopaedic Surgery and Sports Medicine, Harborview Medical Center, University of Washington, 325 9th Avenue, Box 359798, Seattle, WA 98104, USA
* Corresponding author. Harborview Medical Center, 325 Ninth Avenue, Box 359798, Seattle, WA 98104-2499.
E-mail address: daphneb@uw.edu

Orthop Clin N Am 44 (2013) 35–45
http://dx.doi.org/10.1016/j.ocl.2012.08.010
0030-5898/13/$ – see front matter © 2013 Elsevier Inc. All rights reserved.

the lateral column, the articular surface of the distal humerus is the capitellum, which articulates with the radius, to form the radiocapitellar joint. Proximal to the trochlear and capitellar articular surfaces are two concave zones, the olecranon fossa posteriorly and the coronoid fossa anteriorly, which engage the olecranon and coronoid, respectively, during extremes of elbow extension and flexion.

Blood Supply

The blood supply to the elbow is made up primarily of branches of the brachial artery, located anteriorly at the elbow joint. The ulnar and radial collateral branches form an anastomosis with the radial and ulnar recurrent arteries around the joint itself, and these arteries are supplemented by branches from the profunda brachii artery posteriorly. The capitellum receives most of its blood supply posteriorly, which becomes relevant with coronal shear injuries, where posterior stripping should be avoided.

Nerves

The radial, ulnar, and median nerves all cross the elbow joint; however, only the radial and ulnar nerves are typically visualized with fixation of distal humerus fractures via a posterior approach. The ulnar nerve arises from the brachial plexus and travels down the arm in the anterior muscular compartment. The nerve then dives into the posterior compartment at the Arcade of Struthers, approximately 8 cm proximal to the medial epicondyle. It can easily be found closely approximated behind the medial epicondyle, and then it continues through the cubital tunnel and between the two heads of the flexor carpi ulnaris.

The radial nerve leaves the brachial plexus in the posterior compartment of the arm and travels in a distal, lateral path, crossing the humerus approximately 21 cm proximal to the medial and 14 cm proximal to the lateral epicondyle, respectively.[3] The radial nerve lies in the spiral groove of the humerus, closely approximated to bone. Distally it passes through the lateral intramuscular septum approximately 10 cm proximal to the elbow joint.

CLASSIFICATION

There are multiple classification schemes for distal humerus fractures, ranging from descriptive to anatomic. The Arbeitsgemeinschaft für Osteosynthesefragen (AO)/OTA (Orthopaedic Trauma Association) classification is widely used and divides the fractures into types A (extra-articular), B (partial articular), and C (complete articular). In the United Kingdom, 38.7% were found to be type A, 24.1% type B, and 37.2% type C.[4] These types are then subdivided based on extent of comminution and fracture complexity. Another commonly used classification system is that of Jupiter and Mehne which is a descriptive scheme based on the shape of the fracture pattern and its similarity to Roman and Greek alphabet letters.[5]

Capitellar fractures are a specific type of distal humerus fracture with their own classification scheme. In these fractures, a type 1 fracture is a complete capitellar fracture that does not extend into the trochlea; a type 2 fracture consists of an osteochondral fragment that may not have much bony involvement. A type 3 fracture is a comminuted capitellar fracture, and a type 4 fracture is a capitellar fracture that also includes some or all of the trochlea. In this case, a double arc is seen on the lateral radiograph (**Fig. 1**).[6]

INDICATIONS FOR NONOPERATIVE MANAGEMENT

Most distal humerus fractures are treated operatively. On rare occasions, surgeons may elect to treat a distal humerus fracture nonoperatively, which is often related to the patient's overall physiologic status. Indications for nonoperative management include

- Patients who cannot tolerate surgery or those who may not benefit from surgery
- Patients who have neurologic impairment of the limb or overall neurologic impairment.
- Patients with severe osteopenia or bone deficiency
- Patients with soft tissue problems such as local infection or skin loss
- Patients with minimally displaced fractures

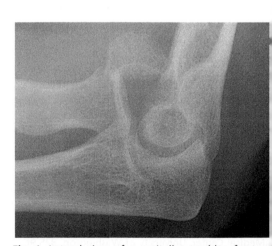

Fig. 1. Lateral view of a capitellar–trochlea fracture demonstrating the double arc sign on the displaced articular fragment, indicating that the fracture fragment includes both capitellum and trochlea.

It is important to note that the risk of stiffness with cast immobilization is high, and this should be weighed against the risks of surgery. Significantly displaced and unstable fractures may be difficult to manage nonoperatively, as they can develop symptomatic nonunions or can cause early problems with pressure areas on the skin, particularly in elderly patients with poor soft tissue quality. As such, fractures distal to the olecranon fossa or coronal shear injuries of the trochlea and capitellum are easier to manage nonoperatively than unstable supracondylar fractures. Careful and vigilant follow-up must be performed if nonoperative management is chosen.

INDICATIONS FOR SURGICAL MANAGEMENT

Any intra-articular fracture of the distal humerus should be considered for surgical management. In rare cases with articular displacement less than 2 mm, these fractures may be managed nonoperatively, as discussed previously, but most of these injuries benefit from open reduction and internal fixation. In addition, associated injuries such as open fractures, concomitant radius and ulna fractures, and neurovascular injuries should point the surgeon toward operative management. Displaced extra-articular (AO/OTA type A) fractures may also be considered for operative management, as controlling reduction of the distal segment in a cast or splint can be difficult and can lead to elbow stiffness. In low-demand patients with osteopenia and very comminuted distal humerus fractures, total elbow arthroplasty is a viable alternative to open reduction and internal fixation. Patients with significant soft tissue defects or contamination can be considered for external fixation as a temporizing measure, although this scenario is uncommon.

PREOPERATIVE EXAMINATION AND PLANNING

In all cases, patients should be completely evaluated for other injuries in addition to the distal humerus fracture. In addition, a complete examination of the upper extremity should be performed, including inspection for open wounds or skin at risk, as well as a neurologic examination including the median, radial, and ulnar nerves, and their more distal branches such as the anterior and posterior interosseous nerves and the cutaneous branches. Almost 25% of patients have preoperative ulnar nerve symptoms in type C distal humerus fractures.[7] Evaluation of radial and ulnar pulses is performed and may be compared with the contralateral arm if any abnormalities are detected.

In addition to elbow and forearm films, anteroposterior (AP) and lateral radiographs of the entire humerus up to the shoulder to evaluate for any proximal extension are obtained. AP and lateral traction radiographs of the elbow are extremely helpful for further delineating the fragments and for preoperative planning. Although computed tomography (CT) scans are sometimes used to evaluate elbow injuries, these views are often not orthogonal to the fracture and may or may not be useful for evaluation of the distal humeral fragments. They are particularly useful in examination of other areas of elbow injury such as the radial head, and they may help further delineate coronal shear injuries of the distal humerus. Three-dimensional reconstructions may be particularly useful in this regard. It is important to note that many patients with distal humeral fractures have other injuries about the elbow, and the surgeon should always search for these to avoid missed diagnoses.

APPROACHES

The patient is positioned either prone or lateral with the shoulder abducted and the elbow flexed to 90° over a radiolucent arm holder. The arm is sterilely prepared and draped up to the axilla. The authors do not routinely use a tourniquet, but a sterile tourniquet should be available in case it becomes necessary during the procedure.

Multiple approaches to the distal humerus have been described.[1] A universal posterior midline skin incision is used, with variations in the deep approach through or around the triceps musculature (**Fig. 2**). The incision should have full-thickness fascio-cutaneous flaps to avoid

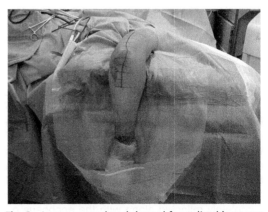

Fig. 2. Arm prepared and draped for a distal humerus fracture repair. The patient is in the lateral position, and a posterior midline incision is marked with the incision line curving radially at the olecranon to avoid wound problems directly over that region.

devascularization of the skin and seroma formation. The incision should be curved over the lateral aspect of the olecranon to facilitate coverage of the hardware at closure and to avoid cutting directly through the olecranon bursa, which may increase hematoma formation.

Olecranon Intact

In cases of minimal articular comminution or extra-articular fracture, a triceps-sparing or triceps-splitting approach may be used. In these approaches, the olecranon is left intact, which decreases ability to visualize the articular surface extensively. These approaches are not recommended for fractures with multiple articular fragments. Since the ulnar nerve is closely approximated to the medial epicondyle, with any approach to the distal humerus it should be identified and dissected to avoid injury. Proximally, the nerve is released along its entirety, including the distal medial intermuscular septum and Osborne ligament to avoid any stretch or tension during the remainder of the surgical procedure. It is also released distally through the extent of the cubital tunnel down to the fascia of the flexor carpi ulnaris to its first motor branch.

Triceps-Sparing

The triceps-sparing approach described by Alonso-Llames[8] is the most commonly used approach. It allows for elevation of the medial and lateral sides of the triceps off the medial and lateral intermuscular septa, respectively. The anconeus is also elevated with the lateral portion of the triceps. The triceps-sparing approach is an excellent option for total elbow arthroplasty, as the olecranon remains intact, and patients can start immediate elbow range of motion without restrictions. This approach can be converted to an olecranon osteotomy if necessary during the procedure (**Fig. 3**).

Bryan-Morrey

A modification of this approach, also known as the Bryan-Morrey approach, allows for complete mobilization of the triceps without detachment.[9] With this approach, a direct posterior incision is made to expose the triceps and olecranon; then the triceps insertion onto the olecranon is elevated subperiosteally starting on the ulnar side. This is completely reflected along with the anconeus on the radial side. At the completion of the procedure, the triceps aponeurosis is repaired through drill holes into the olecranon. The Bryan-Morrey approach is most commonly used for total elbow

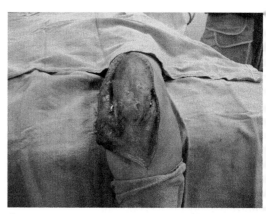

Fig. 3. Triceps-sparing approach working on the medial and lateral side of the triceps. This approach can be easily converted into an olecranon osteotomy by carrying the dissection distally to the subcutaneous border of the olecranon.

arthroplasty and is not easily converted to an olecranon osteotomy.

Triceps-Splitting

The triceps-splitting approach is also known as the Campbell approach.[10] A straight posterior approach is taken to the elbow to expose the triceps. The triceps is then split directly in the midline and peeled subperiosteally to expose the distal humerus. This approach is limited to the distal half of the humeral shaft (approximately 15 cm), as it cannot be extended past the radial nerve and its tethered branches. It is typically used in cases where there is already significant disruption of the triceps by the fracture.

Triceps-Reflecting Anconeus Pedicle

The triceps-reflecting anconeus pedicle approach was described by O'Driscoll and allows for complete detachment and more extensive visualization of the distal humeral articular surface, although still with limitations due to the olecranon being intact.[11] Similar to the Bryan-Morrey approach, the triceps is reflected off the olecranon in continuity with the anconeus. However, in this approach, a V-shaped incision is made to reflect the triceps and anconeus completely off the triceps. At the completion of the procedure, the repair is again made through drill holes in the olecranon.

Transolecranon

It is important to note that all of the previously described approaches give limited visualization of the intra-articular portion of the fracture, as the olecranon is still intact and blocking this area.

The posterior transolecranon approach allows for the best visualization of the articular surface of the distal humerus, but adds possible healing complications of the osteotomy site. The olecranon osteotomy allows for 57% visualization of the articular surface, compared with 35% and 46% for the triceps-splitting and triceps-sparing approaches, respectively.[12] In these cases, the anconeus insertion and origins of the extensor and flexor carpi ulnaris are elevated to expose the olecranon; the triceps attachment is carefully preserved to bone. There is a bare area in the trochlear notch that is nonarticular, and the ideal osteotomy site is located here, approximately 3 cm from the tip of the olecranon. The chevron osteotomy is directed apex distal. The osteotomy should be partially performed with a sagittal saw, but this should not be used to breach the articular surface. The articular surface itself should be breached with an osteotome to create a slightly irregular surface that will interdigitate during fixation. A penrose drain or sponge may be placed in the joint for protection.

Some surgeons advocate predrilling for hardware placement before the osteotomy is made to more anatomically bring the fracture surface together after completion of the procedure (**Fig. 4**). The osteotomy can be repaired in a variety of ways, including a tension band construct consisting of Kirschner wires or a screw-and-tension band or plate-and-screw fixation. Hardware prominence and delayed union or nonunion are the major complications of the olecranon osteotomy.

Lateral Extensile

In isolated capitellar fractures, a lateral extensile approach is recommended. This can be done through either a posterior incision elevating a full-thickness lateral flap or a lateral incision, depending on the need for further fixation around the elbow. The deep incision elevates the wrist extensors and anterior capsule in a full-thickness sleeve anteriorly from the distal humerus. Care is taken to avoid any posterior dissection that could further disrupt the blood supply to the capitellum. The deep incision is continued distally in the Kocher interval between the extensor carpi ulnaris and anconeus.

Ulnar Nerve Transposition

At the conclusion of the procedure, there is some controversy regarding transposition versus simple replacement of the ulnar nerve in the cubital tunnel. A recent study showed that routine ulnar nerve transposition increased postoperative ulnar neuritis.[4] The authors do not routinely transpose

the ulnar nerve, but it is crucial to protect the nerve from contacting metallic implants directly. In addition, the authors take the elbow through a complete range of motion at the conclusion of the procedure to confirm that the nerve is not tethered in any way. If the nerve is tethered or unstable in the tunnel or if the patient has pre-existing ulnar nerve symptoms, a transposition should be considered. In addition, a recent study showed that patients with ulnar nerve symptoms presenting preoperatively may benefit from transposition.[7]

TECHNIQUES FOR FIXATION

As exemplified by the AO, the goal of open reduction and internal fixation (ORIF) in any fracture is to form a stable construct that gives the patient the ability to mobilize quickly. The distal humerus is no exception to this rule. Accurate articular surface reconstruction is crucial for long-term elbow joint function and should decrease the incidence of post-traumatic arthritis.

Fixation Strategies

Once the joint has been exposed in the most appropriate method as chosen by the surgeon, the fracture fragments are completely visualized and cleaned of any debris or hematoma clot that has formed. It is particularly important to pay attention to free-floating fragments and their orientation so that the articular surface can be appropriately reconstructed if these pieces are removed from the field.

In many cases, the articular fragments are first reduced and held provisionally with small (0.035 and 0.045 in) Kirschner, which may be non-threaded or partially threaded to assist with lagging of small fragments (**Fig. 5**). The non-threaded Kirschner wires are particularly useful if the surgeon needs to bury the Kirschner wire in bone on one side before placing a plate, but wishes to remove it from the opposite direction. The articular surface may also be held together using minifragment screws outside the planes of future fixation through plates or with bio-absorbable pegs. Screws heads may be countersunk through the articular surface in coronal plane or shear fractures.

Once the articular surface has been reconstructed, it is then attached back to the shaft at the metaphyseal or diaphyseal area of fracture. Occasionally if one column has a very simple fracture pattern and can be easily used to judge length and alignment of the distal humerus articular surface, this column may be reduced first, and the rest of the articular surface is then reduced to the intact column. During reconstruction of the

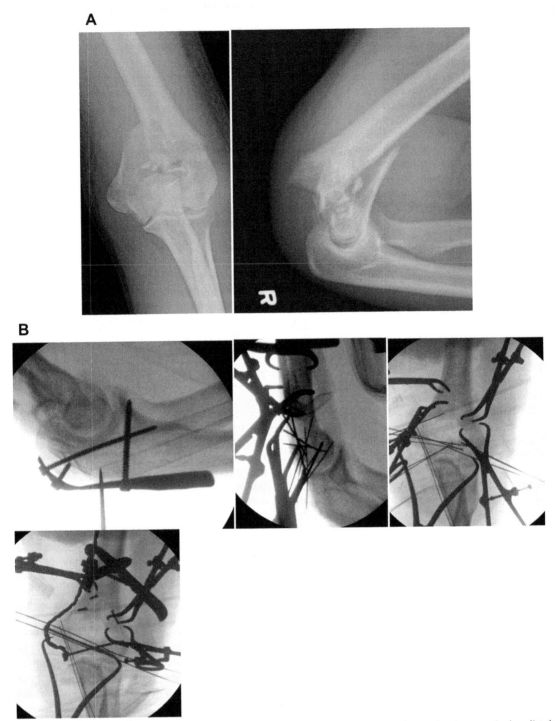

Fig. 4. (*A*) AP and lateral radiograph of a 35-year-old man with a comminuted complex intra-articular distal humerus frature. (*B*) This fracture is best addressed with an olecranon osteotomy. The fixation plate is first pre-drilled with three screws, and the osteotomy location is confirmed with fluoroscopy by placing an osteotome on the dorsal surface of the ulna and marking the area. This exposure allows for anatomic alignment of the articular surface, which is then provisionally secured with Kirschner wires, clamps and minifragment screws to secure the noncomminuted portion of metaphysic. (*C*) The fracture is held with a more flexible 2.7 mm reconstruction plate medially. Note that the trochlea was separated from the medial epicondyle. The plate is contoured medially such that it wraps around the epicondyle, and a screw is placed across the articular segment through the plate. The lateral implant is stiffer than the more flexible medial plate. The osteotomy is anatomically aligned and held with the predrilled plate. (*D*) AP and lateral radiographs taken 3 months postoperatively show a healed fracture and osteotomy.

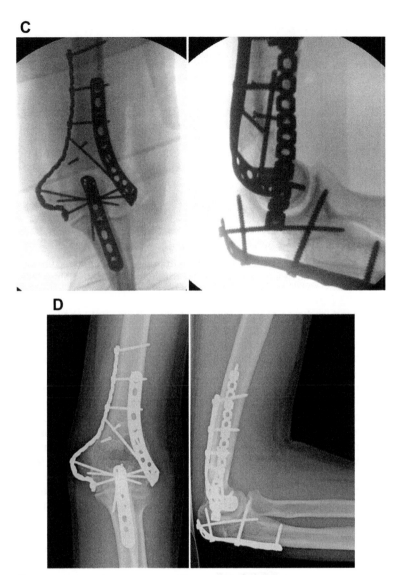

Fig. 4. (*continued*)

articular surface, lag screws are often placed either through or outside of a plate to cross the entire capitellar and trochlear portion of the distal humerus (see **Fig. 4**). If there has been articular cartilage loss in this region, it is very important that the surgeon anatomically restore the width of the distal humerus articular surface and take care not to compress where there has been cartilage loss, which would lead to joint incongruence.

Biomechanical Construct

Multiple constructs have been recommended for fixation of the articular surface to the metaphysic and diaphysis of the humerus. In all cases, authors

note that plates should be placed on each column to augment the screw fixation.[13] Many different plate types have been employed, ranging from 3.5 mm reconstruction plates to 3.5 mm small fragment compression plates. The authors do not recommend one-third tubular plates, as these have been shown to be weaker than necessary for adequate bone stability. In recent years, there have been a number of companies making anatomically contoured distal humeral plates, with both locking and nonlocking options. In these cases, most are 3.5 mm plates, some with smaller distal screws near the articular surface. It is also helpful to have minifragment plates available for provisional fixation in cases where the fracture

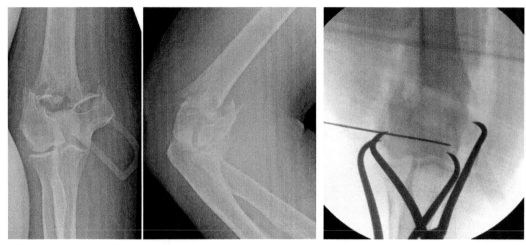

Fig. 5. AP and lateral radiographs of a 67-year-old woman with a distal humerus fracture and a simple articular split. Reduction was obtained through a triceps-sparing approach and held with clamps and Kirschner wires.

fragment has an easily reduced area of bone that may not be easily held with the final plate construct or with provisional wires and clamps (**Fig. 6**).

The primary plate construct has been studied in several articles, and there is still some controversy regarding the supremacy of 90–90 plating (ie, a direct medial plate on the ulnar side of the bone and a direct posterior plate on the radial side of the bone) versus 180° plating (ie, direct medial and direct lateral plates).[13–16] As with most fractures, however, the primary method of gaining stability is an excellent reduction of the fracture itself. In patients with osteopenic bone or bone loss due to comminution or open wounds, locking screws, particularly in the articular portion of the fracture, may augment stability; however,

studies have not shown that locking plates augment a construct in any fracture significantly more than the biomechanical advantages of the 90–90 and 180° plating as described previously.[17] In general, one column should have a more stout plate of 3.5 mm LCDC (Limited Contact Dynamic Compression) thickness, and the other column may be more malleable such as a 3.5 mm or 2.7 mm reconstruction thickness. Since the medial contouring is more complex, the lateral plate is typically the stouter implant (**Fig. 7**). If the trochlea is a separate fragment from the rest of the medial epicondyle, the medial plate should wrap around the medial epicondyle such that a screw can be placed across the articular components through the plate (see **Fig. 4**). Plate placement should be determined by fracture configuration, with plates placed in the most biomechanically sound placement in relation to the fracture lines rather than in positions predetermined by the plate system itself. For fractures distal to the olecranon and coronoid fossa such as transcondylar fractures or coronal shear fractures, less rigid smaller caliber implants are sufficient.

Bone Grafting

In cases of bone loss or comminution, bone grafting may be necessary. Structural autologous graft from the iliac crest is the gold standard for bone grafting; however, there is potential for complications from the bone graft site, and the surgeon may elect to choose allograft instead. Various types exist, from demineralized bone matrix void fillers to structural cortical allograft from donor bone. Each of these bone grafting options should be used at the surgeon's discretion, depending

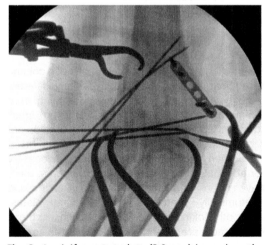

Fig. 6. A minifragment plate (2.0 mm) is used on the medial column to secure the metaphyseal reduction as it was not amenable to clamping.

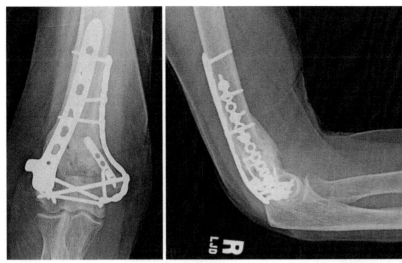

Fig. 7. Radiographs at 5 months demonstrate a healed fracture. Once again, a stiffer lateral implant was used with a more flexible medial implant. The implants were placed at 90° to each other, as that was the optimal placement with respect to the fracture planes.

on the type of bone loss and biomechanical properties deemed necessary at the time of surgery. In rare cases with extensive bone comminution in the metadiaphyseal region, humeral shortening at the fracture site up to 2 cm is acceptable to increase construct stability, especially in patients with osteopenia.[18]

O'Driscoll summarized some technical pearls for surgical fixation of distal humerus fractures[18]:

> Every screw in the distal fragments should pass through a plate.
> Engage a fragment on the opposite side that is also fixed to a plate.
> As many screws as possible should be placed in the distal fragments.
> Each screw should be as long as possible.
> Each screw should engage as many articular fragments as possible.
> The screws in the distal fragments should lock together by interdigitation, creating a fixed-angle structure.
> Plates should be applied such that compression is achieved at the supracondylar level for both columns.
> The plates must be strong enough and stiff enough to resist breaking or bending before union occurs at the supracondylar level.

In cases of isolated coronal shear fractures of the articular surface, countersunk headless screws or bioabsorbable devices are used from an anterior-to-posterior direction, again to preserve the posterior blood supply to this region.[19] If the coronal shear fracture is not isolated, fracture patterns in other planes can be treated as previously described.

Total Elbow Arthroplasty

In elderly or low-demand patients with osteoporosis and severe fracture comminution, or in patients with pre-existing inflammatory arthritis, some studies have shown that a total elbow arthroplasty (TEA) may give better functional outcomes than ORIF of distal humeral fractures (**Fig. 8**).[20] In these studies, there was not a significant difference in complication rates between TEA and ORIF; however, the TEA prosthesis does have some risk of loosening with long-term overuse, and a permanent restriction of weight bearing less than 5 pounds is recommended. In cases where TEA is being considered, the surgeon cannot use an olecranon osteotomy approach; the ulnar component of the arthroplasty uses this bone for fixation, and osteotomy would compromise this area. A triceps-sparing approach is preferable, since it provides adequate space for implant insertion while allowing for immediate postoperative mobilization with no restrictions for triceps healing.

POSTOPERATIVE MANAGEMENT

After ORIF or TEA for a distal humerus fracture, it is important to begin elbow range of motion early to avoid postoperative stiffness. Postoperatively, the authors' patients are placed in a posterior splint in full extension to protect the incision. The splint

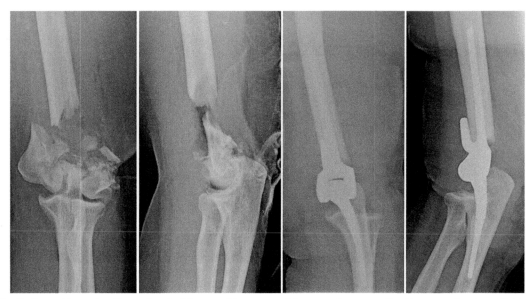

Fig. 8. AP and lateral radiographs of a 75-year-old woman with a complex open distal humerus fracture. She had significant osteopenia, articular comminution, and metaphyseal bone loss. This injury was successfully treated with TEA.

is taken down 48 hours after surgery, and a tubigrip dressing is placed for swelling. Active and active assisted motion of the shoulder and elbow is started. Sutures are left in place for at least 14 days, since healing must occur over a mobile joint surface. Although most regimens focus on regaining extensions, patients are more functionally impaired with activities of daily living early on when they have decreased elbow flexion. As part of their therapy, they are encouraged to use the affected extremity for light activities such as personal hygiene or eating as long as they do not lift anything greater than 1 pound. In patients who have had an olecranon osteotomy, active extension against gravity or resistance is avoided for approximately 6 weeks after fixation. At approximately 6 weeks, patients start more aggressive motion and some strengthening if fracture healing is seen radiographically. By 3 months, patients are working on full strengthening, and at 6 months, they are cleared to return to all activities. If patients have prominent or painful hardware, removal is delayed until approximately 1 year from the time of injury except in rare circumstances.

COMPLICATIONS

The most common complication after distal humerus fracture is stiffness, which is typically present to some degree after fixation. Full extension is the most common area of motion loss. Other complications include fixation failure (most common in one study), superficial wound infections,

nonunion, hardware pain or prominence, contracture, malunion, ulnar or radial nerve palsies, and heterotopic ossification.[21] Heterotopic ossification is another area of controversy, with some authors recommending prophylaxis, such as indomethacin or radiation. Studies show that heterotopic ossification may occur in up to half of patients.[22] However, it may or may not cause functional problems. Risk factors for heterotopic ossification include multiple surgeries and head injury. Routine radiation prophylaxis is not recommended, as it may increase nonunion incidence. In addition, indomethacin treatment may be contraindicated in patients with multiple fractures.

OUTCOMES

Overall outcomes of open reduction and internal fixation of complex distal humerus fractures are satisfactory or better in 71% to 86% of patients.[23] Overall arc of motion of approximately 100° should be expected on average.[24] Patients should also expect approximately 75% return of strength in the distal humeral fracture arm versus their uninjured arm.[24] In osteoporotic, low-demand patients, functional outcomes are similar in ORIF compared with TEA.[25]

REFERENCES

1. Galano GJ, Ahmad CS, Levine WN. Current treatment strategies for bicolumnar distal humerus fractures. J Am Acad Orthop Surg 2010;18(1):20–30.

2. Gray H. Syndesmology: Elbow Joint. In: Lewis WH, editor. Anatomy of the Human body. 20th edition. New York: Bartleby; 1918.

3. Gerwin M, Hotchkiss RN, Weiland AJ. Alternative operative exposures of the posterior aspect of the humeral diaphysis with reference to the radial nerve. J Bone Joint Surg Am 1996;78(11): 1690–5.

4. Chen RC, Harris DJ, Leduc S, et al. Is ulnar nerve transposition beneficial during open reduction internal fixation of distal humerus fractures? J Orthop Trauma 2010;24(7):391–4.

5. Jupiter JB, Mehne DK. Fractures of the distal humerus. Orthopedics 1992;15(7):825–33.

6. McKee MD, Jupiter JB, Bamberger HB. Coronal shear fractures of the distal end of the humerus. J Bone Joint Surg Am 1996;78(1):49–54.

7. Ruan HJ, Liu JJ, Fan CY, et al. Incidence, management, and prognosis of early ulnar nerve dysfunction in type C fractures of distal humerus. J Trauma 2009; 67(6):1397–401.

8. Alonso-Llames M. Bilaterotricipital approach to the elbow. Its application in the osteosynthesis of supracondylar fractures of the humerus in children. Acta Orthop Scand 1972;43(6):479–90.

9. Bryan RS, Morrey BF. Extensive posterior exposure of the elbow. A triceps-sparing approach. Clin Orthop Relat Res 1982;(166):188–92.

10. Anglen J. Distal humerus fractures. J Am Acad Orthop Surg 2005;13(5):291–7.

11. O'Driscoll SW. The triceps-reflecting anconeus pedicle (TRAP) approach for distal humeral fractures and nonunions. Orthop Clin North Am 2000; 31(1):91–101.

12. Wilkinson JM, Stanley D. Posterior surgical approaches to the elbow: a comparative anatomic study. J Shoulder Elbow Surg 2001;10(4):380–2.

13. Helfet DL, Hotchkiss RN. Internal fixation of the distal humerus: a biomechanical comparison of methods. J Orthop Trauma 1990;4(3):260–4.

14. Zalavras CG, Vercillo MT, Jun BJ, et al. Biomechanical evaluation of parallel versus orthogonal plate fixation of intra-articular distal humerus fractures. J Shoulder Elbow Surg 2011;20(1):12–20.

15. Penzkofer R, Hungerer S, Wipf F, et al. Anatomical plate configuration affects mechanical performance in distal humerus fractures. Clin Biomech (Bristol, Avon) 2010;25(10):972–8.

16. Kollias CM, Darcy SP, Reed JG, et al. Distal humerus internal fixation: a biomechanical comparison of 90 degrees and parallel constructs. Am J Orthop (Belle Mead NJ) 2010;39(9):440–4.

17. Korner J, Diederichs G, Arzdorf M, et al. A biomechanical evaluation of methods of distal humerus fracture fixation using locking compression plates versus conventional reconstruction plates. J Orthop Trauma 2004;18(5):286–93.

18. O'Driscoll SW. Optimizing stability in distal humeral fracture fixation. J Shoulder Elbow Surg 2005; 14(1 Suppl S):186S–94S.

19. Mehdian H, McKee MD. Fractures of capitellum and trochlea. Orthop Clin North Am 2000;31(1):115–27.

20. Burkhart KJ, Nijs S, Mattyasovszky SG, et al. Distal humerus hemiarthroplasty of the elbow for comminuted distal humeral fractures in the elderly patient. J Trauma 2011;71(3):635–42.

21. Sodergard J, Sandelin J, Bostman O. Postoperative complications of distal humeral fractures. 27/96 adults followed up for 6 (2–10) years. Acta Orthop Scand 1992;63(1):85–9.

22. Eralp L, Kocaoglu M, Sar C, et al. Surgical treatment of distal intra-articular humeral fractures in adults. Int Orthop 2001;25(1):46–50.

23. Frattini M, Soncini G, Corradi M, et al. Midterm results of complex distal humeral fractures. Musculoskelet Surg 2011;95(3):205–13.

24. O'Driscoll SW, Jupiter JB, Cohen MS, et al. Difficult elbow fractures: pearls and pitfalls. Instr Course Lect 2003;52:113–34.

25. Egol KA, Tsai P, Vazques O, et al. Comparison of functional outcomes of total elbow arthroplasty vs plate fixation for distal humerus fractures in osteoporotic elbows. Am J Orthop (Belle Mead NJ) 2011; 40(2):67–71.

Terrible Triad of the Elbow

Seth D. Dodds, MD*, Thomas Fishler, MD

KEYWORDS

- Terrible triad • Elbow • Ulnohumeral • Radiocapitellar • Proximal radioulnar

KEY POINTS

- The elbow is a 3-dimensionally complex joint where stiffness is poorly tolerated and instability is devastating.
- Although multiple periarticular fracture patterns and soft tissue injuries of the elbow have been described, the combination of coronoid process fracture, radial head fracture, and elbow dislocation has earned the moniker "terrible triad" by virtue of its challenging treatment and historically poor outcomes.
- This injury represents a failure of each bony and ligamentous stabilizer of the elbow; therefore, treatment must restore sufficient stability to permit early motion, thereby avoiding disabling stiffness.

INTRODUCTION

The elbow is a 3-dimensionally complex joint where stiffness is poorly tolerated and instability is devastating. Although multiple periarticular fracture patterns and soft tissue injuries of the elbow have been described, the combination of coronoid process fracture, radial head fracture, and elbow dislocation has earned the moniker "terrible triad" by virtue of its challenging treatment and historically poor outcomes.[1–5] This injury represents a failure of each bony and ligamentous stabilizer of the elbow; therefore, treatment must restore sufficient stability to permit early motion, thereby avoiding disabling stiffness.

RELEVANT ANATOMY

The elbow supports the intersection of 3 bones, between which are 3 articulations: ulnohumeral, radiocapitellar, and proximal radioulnar (**Fig. 1**). The first two of these articulations are ginglymus (hinge) joints, whereas the last is a trochoid (pivot) joint. The terrible triad injury destabilizes the relationship between the humerus and the forearm bones, whereas the relationship between the ulna and radius (including the interosseous membrane) is rarely disrupted in this injury pattern.

While the elbow shares the humerus in common with the shoulder joint, its personality could not possibly be more different. Unlike the relatively straightforward spheroidal glenohumeral joint with its complex circumferential soft tissue stabilizers, the elbow has a complex three-dimensional bony anatomy but relatively simple soft tissue structure consisting of medial and lateral collateral ligaments as well as anterior and posterior capsular elements.

The trochlea of the distal humerus is located centrally, in line with the shaft of the humerus, and articulates with the greater sigmoid notch of the proximal ulna. The apex of the trochlea articulates with the sagittal ridge of the greater sigmoid notch, making the ulnohumeral joint a highly congruent and inherently stable articulation.[6]

The radiocapitellar joint is also a hinge but has much less intrinsic stability. Nevertheless, it functions as an important stabilizer of the elbow against valgus stress. The radial head is elliptical, so as to allow the bicipital tuberosity to not impinge on the ulna when the forearm is in full pronation, but this elliptical shape is not consistent between individuals.[7,8] The anterior and posterior capsules are relatively uniform, without discrete thickenings. Laterally and medially, however, distinct thickenings form the collateral ligament complexes, each of which is composed of multiple components.

Hand and Upper Extremity Surgery, Department of Orthopaedics and Rehabilitation, Yale University School of Medicine, 800 Howard Avenue, Yale Physician's Building 133, New Haven, CT 06519, USA
* Corresponding author.
E-mail address: seth.dodds@yale.edu

Orthop Clin N Am 44 (2013) 47–58
http://dx.doi.org/10.1016/j.ocl.2012.08.006

orthopedic.theclinics.com

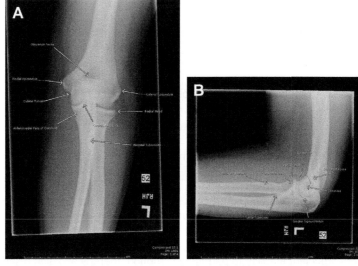

Fig. 1. Bony landmarks as seen on (A) anteroposterior (AP) and (B) lateral radiographs.

The medial collateral ligament (MCL) complex is composed of 3 bands: anterior, posterior, and transverse (**Fig. 2**A). The first two originate from the inferior aspect of the medial epicondyle, whereas the last one does not cross the elbow joint itself. The anterior band is the most distinct and significant of these bundles and inserts on the sublime tubercle of the coronoid. Inserting more posteriorly, on the olecranon, is the posterior band, whereas the transverse band is attached at both ends to the ulna, spanning the distance from the tip of the olecranon to the coronoid process.

Laterally, the collateral ligament complex is similarly made of up of 3 components: the lateral ulnar collateral ligament (LUCL), the radial collateral ligament, and the annular ligament (see **Fig. 2**B). Similar to the MCL complex, the first two components attach proximally on the epicondyle, whereas the annular ligament is a proximal radioulnar joint stabilizer that both originates and inserts on the ulna. The LUCL, which inserts on the crista supinatoris of the posterior proximal ulna, is a major stabilizer against varus stress and also supports the radial head like a sling, preventing posterolateral rotatory subluxation. The radial collateral ligament does not attach to the radius or ulna directly, but rather to the annular ligament.

BIOMECHANICS

Load bearing across the elbow is predominantly at the radiocapitellar joint (60%), rather than at the ulnohumeral joint (40%).[9] The latter, with its highly congruent configuration, is structured primarily for stability rather than for load bearing and contributes as much as 50% of the overall stability of the elbow.[10] The stability conferred by these bony structures is what allows most simple elbow dislocations to remain stable after reduction.[11] As displacing forces most commonly act

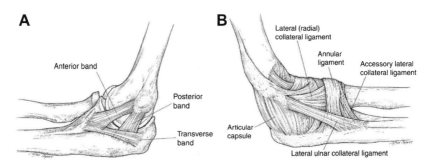

Fig. 2. Ligamentous stabilizers of the elbow. (A) The medial collateral ligament. (B) The lateral collateral ligament complex. (*Reproduced from* Bain GI, Mehta JA. Anatomy of the elbow joint and surgical approaches. In: Baker Jr, CL, Plancher KD, editors. Operative treatment of elbow injuries. New York: Springer-Verlag; 2001. p. 9–10; with permission.)

on the elbow in a posteriorly directed manner, the coronoid is particularly vital. Large coronoid fragments destabilize the elbow considerably[12,13] and even very small fractures may portend a great deal of instability by virtue of their unique anatomic shape and attachment to the anterior capsule.[14] The latter are more common with terrible triad patterns. Fractures of the anteromedial coronoid are associated with a different mechanism of injury and are uncommon in terrible triad injuries.[15]

As mentioned above, the ulnohumeral and radiocapitellar articulations are hinge joints, but their axis of flexion/extension varies with position,[16–18] by approximately 3° to 6° in orientation and 1.4 to 2.0 mm in translation.[19] On average, however, this axis runs from the anteroinferior aspect of the medial epicondyle (just anterior to the origin of the anterior band of the MCL) to the center of the trochlea and the center of the capitellum on lateral radiography. The location of this axis has important implications for the placement of hinged external fixators in particular. Normal range of motion in this plane is 0° to 140° of flexion, although most activities of daily living may be performed with a limited range of 30° to 130°.

Forearm rotation normally encompasses an arc of 180°, divided equally between pronation and supination, although a loss of 30° at either end is usually well tolerated and permits typical activities of daily living.[16,17] Abduction at the shoulder does compensate for limited pronation, but no similar compensatory movement can substitute for supination.[20] Forearm rotation also affects elbow stability. For example, supination of the elbow increases the joint reactive force at the ulnohumeral joint and increases stability against elbow dislocation. However, in the LUCL-deficient elbow, supination is also implicated in posterolateral rotatory instability, whereby the radial head subluxates posterolaterally, whereas the ulna tilts apex lateral.[21] A position of pronation protects against this posterolateral rotatory instability.

In response to valgus stress, the radial head abuts the capitellum and provides approximately 30% of total elbow stability in this scenario, more so when the MCL is incompetent.[22,23] Restoration of the radial head restores valgus stability to nearly that of the intact elbow. The MCL, with its anterior band taut in extension and its posterior band taut in flexion, also resists valgus stress throughout the range of elbow motion.[6]

The lateral collateral ligament (LCL) complex is hypothesized to be the first structure to fail in dislocation of the elbow.[24] The LUCL, as described above, is necessary to prevent posterolateral rotatory instability, and it is the major soft tissue stabilizer of the elbow, against varus stress.

Although there is some controversy as to the exact contribution of each element of the LCL complex,[25–30] it has been demonstrated that reconstruction of the LUCL alone reliably restores posterolateral stability,[31] suggesting that LUCL is the primary critical stabilizer against this particular instability pattern.

The terrible triad injury pattern most commonly results from the axial loading of a relatively extended elbow with the forearm in supination (**Fig. 3**). This position encourages posterolateral escape of the radial head after failure of the LUCL, whereas the axial loading causes shearing of the radial head and coronoid process. In fact, the terrible triad can be conceptualized quite accurately as the *ultimate* posterolateral rotatory instability.

PRESENTATION

The terrible triad is an injury of the adult elbow. The mechanism may be either high or low energy. In Ring's series of 22 patients, 12 occurred as a result of a fall from standing, with the remaining 10 caused by a fall from a greater height.[32] In Mckee's series of 40 patients, 14 were attributed to falls from standing, 11 to higher energy falls, 5 to bicycle accidents, 4 to sports injuries, and 1 each to motorcycle accident and crush injury.[33]

Typically, the most obvious component of the injury is dislocation of the elbow. However, spontaneous reduction may prevent radiographic documentation of frank instability. A thorough history can reveal such an episode, or alternatively, dislocation can be inferred in the presence

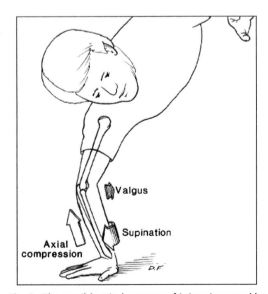

Fig. 3. The terrible triad pattern of injury is caused by a combination of valgus and axial compression with the forearm supinated.

IMAGING

of hallmark fractures of the radial head and coronoid. Nerve involvement, particularly of the ulnar nerve, must be rigorously elicited and documented, after a closed reduction if need be. The presence of ulnar nerve symptoms may dictate whether or not a medial surgical approach is anticipated, as will be discussed later.

IMAGING

Standard anteroposterior (AP) and lateral radiography should be performed as part of the initial evaluation. Oblique radiographs may better characterize a radial head or coronoid fracture pattern. The AP image should also be carefully scrutinized for a fleck of bone off of the lateral epicondyle, representing a bony avulsion of the LUCL. In exceptional circumstances, when the dislocated status of the joint is identifiable on physical examination and a qualified provider is immediately available, closed reduction of the elbow may be performed before standard imaging studies are performed; otherwise, both injury and postreduction images should be evaluated for bony fragments, which can frequently be subtle findings.

Although careful examination of plain radiographs is invaluable, the overlap of the proximal ulna and proximal radius on lateral radiography, as well as the overlap of the coronoid process on the trochlea on AP radiographs, means that conventional radiographs may obscure significant bony injuries. Computed tomography (CT) has been used extensively and effectively as an adjunct imaging modality. However, as with fractures of the distal humerus and proximal ulna, universally accepted indications for CT imaging of terrible triad injuries have not been produced. The authors see CT to be most helpful in identifying occult fractures of the coronoid and/or radial head when such injuries are suspected but not visualized on plain radiographs. In such circumstances, CT findings can change the management profoundly, from closed treatment to open surgery. CT scan has also been identified as a critical imaging modality to assess and characterize the size and morphology of coronoid

fractures[34] and radial head articular fragmentation. Both the size of the coronoid fracture and the degree of articular fragmentation of the radial head alter operative fixation techniques and should be well understood preoperatively.

ACUTE MANAGEMENT

After a thorough history taking and physical examination, closed reduction of the elbow should be performed. An immediate postreduction examination defining the stable range of motion is helpful when fractures of the radial head and coronoid have not been identified on injury radiographs. When the terrible triad injury pattern has already been diagnosed based on initial radiographs, this postreduction assessment may cause additional harm to the already damaged articular surfaces.

A posterior splint is applied with the forearm in neutral position and the elbow reduced in a position of approximately 90° of flexion. While the instability conferred by the terrible triad injury pattern is such that reduction rarely requires extreme effort, soft tissue interposition can occasionally be a block to reduction and fracture fragments may become incarcerated, leading to an incongruous reduction (Fig. 4). A failed reduction demands consideration for either a repeat attempt using (1) closed means and a general anesthetic if the initial attempt was under conscious sedation or (2) an open reduction to clear interposed soft tissues or incarcerated fracture fragments.

After achieving reduction, most terrible triad injuries can be adequately held reduced in a splint, with definitive management scheduled on an elective basis. However, if the reduction is unstable, and the surgeon or circumstances (staff, equipment, etc.) are not optimal for acute definitive management, the elbow may be temporarily stabilized, with a static external fixator or transarticular fixation.

DEFINITIVE MANAGEMENT

Stabilization of the terrible triad using internal means should, as with any complex periarticular

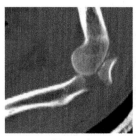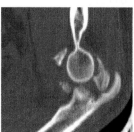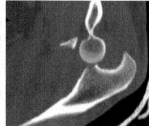

Fig. 4. Incarceration of bony fragments blocking reduction.

racture, be carefully planned and performed under optimal conditions. A rested and familiar staff is beneficial. Despite appropriate planning, many decisions affecting implant choice are made intraoperatively. The necessary equipment for stabilization of a terrible triad elbow is listed n **Box 1**.

The goal of surgical treatment is to restore stability to the ulnohumeral and radiocapitellar oints, allowing early flexion/extension and prono-supination and avoiding crippling stiffness. In the most successful case series in the literature, coronoid and radial head fractures as well as the soft tissue stabilizers of the elbow were addressed.[32,33] Therefore, we recommend addressing all 3 elements of the terrible triad injury in all cases rather than addressing just 1 or 2 and hinging decisions for further stabilizing measures on intraoperative assessment of stability with dynamic fluoroscopy.

Exposure, then, must be extensive enough to allow access to the coronoid, radial head, and collateral ligaments. The radial head and LUCL are both lateral structures that are, naturally, best accessed laterally. The MCL is a medial structure that can only be exposed medially. It is the coronoid that represents a quandary; being more midline than medial in the coronal plane, its key feature is how anterior it is located. Therefore, it may be approached either medially or even laterally. Regardless, the challenge in its exposure comes from the overlying brachialis and flexor–pronator mass, as well as the close proximity of the median nerve and bifurcating brachial artery. Last, it is worth mentioning an injured ulnar nerve, which for reasons other than stability may need

exposure and release, both of which are possible only with a medial approach.

The possibility of needing simultaneous access to the medial as well as the lateral elbow has led some surgeons to recommend a midline posterior skin incision, the so-called global approach to the elbow.[32,33] Skin flaps are then raised medially and laterally until the appropriate deep dissection can be performed on both sides. This utilitarian approach permits full exposure of the elbow and provides a window for revision surgery, such as a capsular release.

The authors use a single lateral skin incision, accompanied by a separate medial incision if required for coronoid exposure, MCL repair, or ulnar nerve transposition. This approach has been popularized by King.[33] The lateral approach is ideal for supine positioning with a fluoroscopically compatible hand table extension. The incision is typically centered over the lateral epicondyle. Distally, the incision is carried out in line with the radius. Once the fascia overlying the extensors is exposed, multiple options exist for deep dissection, including intervals between the extensor carpi radialis longus (ECRL)/extensor carpi radialis brevis (ECRB) and extensor digitorum communis (EDC) (Kaplan) or the extensor carpi ulnaris (ECU) and anconeus (Kocher). The former is marked by a fat stripe visible through the extensor fascia (**Fig. 5**). It has 3 distinct advantages over the ECU–anconeus approach. First, it allows the surgeon to stay anterior to the main substance of the LUCL, without violating it. In this approach, the annular ligament must be divided, but this is a proximal radioulnar joint stabilizer and not a radiocapitellar stabilizer.

Box 1
Equipment for a terrible triad

Hand table

Large fluoroscope

Sterile tourniquet

Surgical headlight

Hand set

2.4- and 2.7-mm screws

Mini fragment plates

Radial head arthroplasty

Hinged elbow external fixator

No. 2 braided nonabsorbable suture

Hewson suture passer

Suture anchors

Semitendinosus allograft

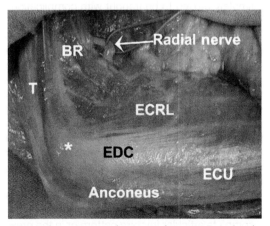

Fig. 5. The extensor fascia. A fat stripe marks the interval between the wrist extensors (ECRL and underlying ECRB) and the common finger extensor. The brachioradialis (BR) and triceps (T) are marked for orientation.

Second, the more anterior approach allows better access to the anterolateral radial head, which is key in the prevention of posterior dislocation.[32] Last, because of the quite anterior location of the coronoid, highlighted previously, the more anterior approach to the radial head also makes for an easier coronoid exposure from the lateral side. Despite these advantages, the principle of working through traumatic intervals should remain a guide; frequently, the injury itself will present the surgeon with a workable plane that requires minimal further insult to the soft tissues.

The exact nature of the injury to the LUCL will be readily apparent early in this exposure. Avulsion of the LUCL off the inferior aspect of the lateral epicondyle is commonplace in these injuries and should be expected. The radial head injury should be thoroughly inspected. Usually, but not always, a preoperative CT scan will reveal all that is important in making the decision between fracture repair and prosthetic replacement. Unexpected comminution or other difficulty has led historically to intraoperative changes in course from repair to arthroplasty in 20% to 40% of cases in which the former was planned.[34] This seemingly low threshold for abandoning open reduction/internal fixation (ORIF) in favor of arthroplasty reflects the implant-driven history of radial head fracture management. Although radial head excision had historically been the standard in operative treatment of these fractures, the development of Arbeitsgemeinschaft fur Osteosynthesefragen (AO) stable internal fixation dramatically increased the popularity of ORIF techniques, and the AO case series of Heim promoted these techniques for all operated fractures.[35] Meanwhile, silicone radial head prostheses, which had been primarily used for nontraumatic indications, ultimately proved to be fraught with complications such as fracture and synovitis.[18,36] Later, biomechanical studies demonstrated that silicone implants are unable to resist valgus stresses in a manner similar to the native radial head.[18,37] The development of metallic radial head replacements revolutionized radial head fracture treatment, with consistently good results reported in the challenging setting of elbow instability and unstable fracture patterns.[32,38-41] At the same time, ORIF of more complex radial head fractures was increasingly shown to be fraught with high complication rates, including early failure of fixation and nonunion.[42-44]

We recommend arthroplasty rather than ORIF in the presence more than 3 articular fragments in a complete articular fracture pattern or in the presence of multiple small irreparable fragments in a partial articular pattern, where those fragments amount to a significant loss of the anterolateral radial head. Extensive impaction of the articular surface is also a relative indication for arthroplasty, as is a concomitant Essex-Lopresti lesion, in which forces on the chosen construct are expected to be higher. If arthroplasty is elected, the radial head should be excised immediately because this will enhance the lateral exposure of the coronoid. If a medial approach is selected, the surgeon is presented with multiple options as to deep dissection. However, when comparing a flexor carpi ulnaris splitting approach to the Hotchkiss "over-the-top" approach,[45] which splits the flexor–pronator mass to approach the coronoid from directly anterior, Huh and colleagues[46] found that the flexor carpi ulnaris (FCU) split better visualized the sublime tubercle and MCL. These approaches can be combined as needed if anterior coronoid fixation and MCL reconstruction are desired. Fractures of the anteromedial coronoid facet, which are caused by varus loading mechanism and are thus rarely seen in terrible triad patterns, can be approached by this same FCU splitting approach.

The coronoid process, located centrally in the coronal plane, is not only the most challenging aspect of terrible triad management but also the key to elbow stability. Exposure of the coronoid from a lateral approach is facilitated by but does not necessitate the excision of the radial head. Most challenging is the exposure of the coronoid in the presence of a partial articular radial head fracture that is to be fixed. The intact portion of the radial head and neck obstructs not only visualization of the coronoid but also direct reduction of the proximal radioulnar joint (PRUJ) portion of the coronoid fracture. In addition, as long as the intact portion of the partial articular fracture of the radial head is located, lateral column length obligates a certain degree of soft tissue tension, which prevents adequate retraction and visualization of the coronoid from the lateral side. In these circumstances, forced supination of the forearm can bring the radial head out posterolaterally, through the failed LUCL, easing tension on the anterior soft tissues and easing exposure of the coronoid. Alternatively, a more generous proximal release of the origin of the brachioradialis and ECRL off the lateral column of the distal humerus will allow for excellent exposure of the anterior tip of the coronoid, looking down from a proximal and lateral vantage point. A surgeon's headlight effectively illuminates poorly visible coronoid fragments within this deep surgical field.

The coronoid fragment may be of any size, but most commonly, it represents 30% to 50% of the total coronoid height.[15] In the authors' case series presented below, the average coronoid height was measured to be 7.6 mm on preoperative CT

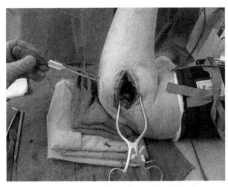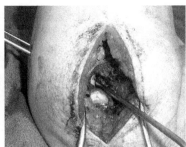

Fig. 6. Screw fixation of the coronoid fragment through a counterincision over the dorsal ulna.

scans. At this size, screw fixation is certainly challenging but possible with careful technique. Posteroanterior screws may be placed through a small counterincision over the subcutaneous border of the proximal ulna (**Fig. 6**). A 2.0-mm drill bit is used in preparation for a 2.7-mm screw. It is helpful to displace the fracture while passing the drill to directly visualize its trajectory at the fracture site. The drill bit can then be withdrawn slightly, the fracture reduced and compressed with a dental pick, and the drill bit advanced through the coronoid tip fracture fragment. After measuring (typical length is approximately 36–40 mm), the screw is inserted while maintaining compression across the fracture site. Occasionally, a coronoid fragment will be wide enough to accept 2 screws. If such a construct is planned, the 2 drill bits should be inserted and left in situ before any screw is placed, to provide provisional rotational stability. An anterior cruciate ligament (ACL) guide or other similar guide may be helpful to facilitate drill bit direction, but these guides may not be accommodated by the anterior soft tissues around the elbow. From a biomechanical perspective, the stability of screw fixation depends on screw head incarceration of the near cortex and far cortical thread purchase; this implies that screws directed AP may achieve a firmer hold on the small coronoid fragment. However, insertion through an anterior stab wound can threaten iatrogenic neurovascular injury; even with an open anterior approach, religious use of a drill guide and oscillation mode is recommended.

Smaller coronoid fracture fragments were once considered stable capsular "avulsions"; this is now well recognized as a misnomer because the mechanism of injury is in fact shear. The anterior elbow capsule inserts some 5.9 mm distal to the tip of the coronoid on average[14] and will typically retain its attachment even in small coronoid fractures. If these fragments are too small to capture with a screw, a soft tissue repair of the anterior capsule provides adequate stability.[47] Heavy nonabsorbable suture is passed through the capsular tissue close to its insertion on the coronoid fragment and then either passed through drill holes in or around the proximal ulna or tied down to the coronoid fracture bed with a suture anchor. Not uncommonly, suture repair may result in an overtightening of the anterior capsule, preventing full extension of the elbow. However, a disabling lack of full extension has a relatively straightforward surgical solution in the form of a staged capsular release after interval healing, whereas residual instability due to inadequate or loose repair leads to more complicated and onerous (for both the surgeon and the patient) treatment with hinged external fixation. A biomechanical cadaver study by Beingessner and colleagues[48] calls into question the stability conferred by repair of small coronoid fragments by soft tissue techniques, but the clinical importance of these findings has yet to be demonstrated. We therefore recommend fixation of all coronoid fractures in the setting of the terrible triad injuries, including small ones, by the bony and soft tissue techniques described above.

After addressing the coronoid, attention is again turned to the radial head. If fracture repair is elected, small implants are essential (**Fig. 7**). In partial articular patterns, only screws or a buttress plate may be used; although the latter is superior biomechanically, the inability to countersink a plate may preclude its use if the fracture involves aspects of the radial head that articulate with the lesser sigmoid notch of the ulna. In complete articular patterns, the articular surface is typically reconstructed first, before metadiaphyseal reduction and fixation. The articular reconstruction itself may even be performed on the back table (see **Fig. 7**C), although if significant soft tissue attachments remain to even one of the articular fragments, this type of devascularization should be avoided.

If arthroplasty is planned, the fractured radial head should have been excised previously to

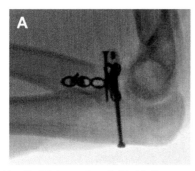
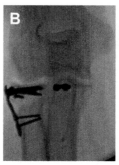
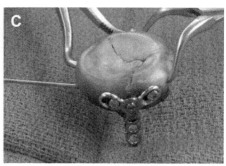

Fig. 7. (*A*) Lateral and (*B*) AP fluoroscopic images of a radial head fracture treated with ORIF. In the case of a complete articular fracture, a back table reconstruction (*C*) may be necessary.

improve coronoid exposure. In the case of partial articular fractures, a neck cut will need to be made. The amount of neck resection necessary will depend on the prosthesis chosen. Regardless, the safety of the posterior interosseous nerve (PIN) must be ensured while extending dissection distally. Although pronation of the forearm is conventionally thought to move this nerve farther from the operative field, a recent cadaveric study looking specifically at the PIN in the setting of radial neck fracture found that the presence of a fracture reduces this protective benefit.[49] Therefore, if there are concerns as to the safety of the PIN, one should directly visualize and protect it (**Fig. 8**).

Metallic radial head prostheses, which have rapidly replaced their silicone equivalents as the gold standard, are available in monoblock and modular designs. Multiple case series have been published to support the clinical outcomes of both monoblock[39,50] and modular[51–53] prostheses. The latter obviously bear a greater cost, but from a technical standpoint, the authors have found that insertion of a radial head of the appropriate diameter is easier with a modular implant. Such an implant allows the prosthesis to be gently implanted without excess stress on what too frequently could be a tenuous coronoid repair.

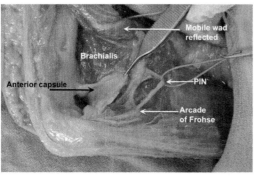

Fig. 8. The PIN is at risk as dissection around the radial neck proceeds distally.

More importantly, it allows the implantation of a radial head with a relatively large diameter but a relatively short neck (**Fig. 9**). The larger diameter head augments stability by better tensioning the lateral ligamentous complex, whereas the short neck avoids radiocapitellar "overstuffing," which leads to capitellar erosion.[54]

Precisely defining a consistently reliable method to size the radial head has proved to be an enduring problem. Doornberg and colleagues[55] attempted to describe reference points based on the coronoid process, but these were stymied by the significant variability between patients that they discovered. On this basis, contralateral radiographs were chosen by Athwal and colleagues[56] to judge over-lengthening in a group of patients and predict radial head prosthesis size in a cadaveric group. In the latter, this method was successfully predictive of prosthesis size 87% of the time. The usefulness of these results to the index surgeon treating an acute terrible triad injury is unknown at this time.

Repair of the lateral soft tissue stabilizers is the last element for most terrible triad procedures. The LUCL, as discussed previously, is most commonly avulsed from the lateral epicondyle as an intact sleeve, giving the surgeon the opportunity for a stout repair as long as firm bony fixation is achieved, which is possible through either bone tunnels or suture anchors. Although the latter incur implant costs, the authors have found anchors to be more user friendly and more precise in bringing the ligament to its anatomic footprint (**Fig. 10**). Suture should be heavy gauge and nonabsorbable, and a locking pattern is preferable. The authors make sure to bury potentially irritating knots within a tightly repaired extensor fascia.

At this stage of the operation, a thorough examination of the elbow for stability is performed with fluoroscopy. A full range of flexion and extension is not necessary, and full extension may in fact lead to disruption of coronoid fracture or anterior capsular repairs. Assessing motion through the

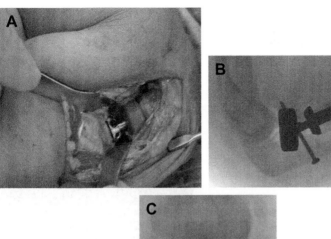

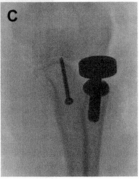

Fig. 9. Prosthetic replacement of the radial head with a modular implant, following coronoid repair. (*A*) Clinical photograph showing the radial neck after in situ lengthening. (*B*) Lateral and (*C*) AP fluoroscopic images showing maintenance of coronoid fixation and a congruent ulnohumeral joint.

functional range from 30° to 130° of flexion suffices. Extra care must be taken to carefully examine the ulnohumeral articulation for congruence. A subtle incongruence along with posterior sagging of the radial head suggests an inadequate lateral soft tissue repair, with resultant posterolateral rotatory instability. Repair or reconstruction of the MCL is a treatment option for residual instability of the ulnohumeral articulation. Routine repair of the MCL is not necessary in light of the impressive results of Forthman and colleagues.[32] In their study, of 34 patients treated with the above-described terrible triad repair and no repair of the MCL, only 2 experienced late instability, with these failures attributed to noncompliance. A similar protocol was followed by McKee,[33] who had just 1 case of persistent instability out of 40 patients.

As an alternative to MCL repair, a hinged or static external fixator may be applied. Augmenting fracture repairs with external fixation, however, carries

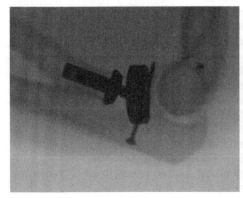

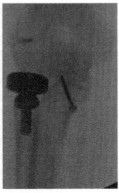

Fig. 10. The final construct, after repairing the lateral ligamentous complex using a suture anchor in the lateral epicondyle.

additional morbidity and is not our preferred option for index treatment. Nonetheless, situations certainly arise in which there is persistent elbow instability. Hinged external fixation needs to be done precisely in order to permit early range of motion. Alternatively, a static external fixator from the humerus anteriorly to the distal third of the dorsal radial shaft (forearm pronated and elbow flexed to 90°) provides excellent stability to an unstable fracture. Such a motion-blocking construct must be either removed or revised to a hinged device within 3 weeks, to avoid irrecoverable loss of motion.

POSTOPERATIVE CARE

While early motion is crucial to avoiding stiffness-related complications, protection in a splint, with the elbow at 90° of flexion, eases pain control and encourages wound healing. An early follow-up in the surgeon's clinic is a must, giving the surgeon the opportunity to check the wound, educate the patient, and initiate motion. The authors' postoperative protocol involves initiation of motion at 2 weeks after surgery after radiographs confirm maintenance of a concentric reduction. Patients begin flexion exercises first to regain the ability to bring the hand to mouth. Forearm rotation may also be done with the elbow at 90°. At 3 weeks after surgery, patients begin active elbow extension. If there are concerns for instability, elbow extension with the patient supine and the forearm pronated stabilizes the elbow and minimize stress on LCL repair. Lastly, frequent radiographs are recommended to ensure concentric ulnohumeral and radiocapitellar joint reductions during the healing process, especially as the therapy progresses.

OUTCOMES

The largest series of terrible triad injuries treated with the current standard surgical treatment of coronoid ORIF, radial head ORIF or arthroplasty, and LUCL repair have been published by Ring[32] (22 patients) and McKee[33] (40 patients). In the former series, average arc of motion was 17° to 117°, with the average Broberg and Morrey score being 88. In the latter series, 1 patient had late instability requiring application of a hinged external fixator, with the mean Mayo Elbow Performance Score also being 88.

In the authors' own series of 15 patients with follow-up available, the average arc of motion was 26° to 132°, with the average Mayo Elbow Score being 85. A total of 2 patients had poor outcomes, both of whom were patients with polytrauma. Of these, 1 had closed head injuries that

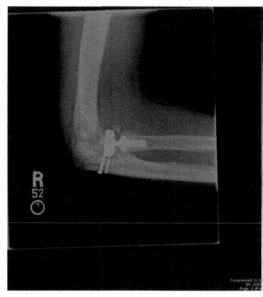

Fig. 11. Heterotopic ossification causing stiffness. This patient went on to surgical excision and radical release.

delayed rehabilitation, leading to stiffness and heterotopic ossification (**Fig. 11**) necessitating radical release. The other patient had bilateral pilon fractures, necessitating aggressive early mobilization of her upper extremity; she ultimately went on to show signs of residual instability.

COMPLICATIONS

The most feared complication of the terrible triad injury is persistent instability, which, in a joint as prone to stiffness as the elbow, has no good solution. Late instability can be managed by hinged external fixation, augmented by LUCL reconstruction with a tendon graft in select circumstances.[57] Forthman and colleagues[32] saw this complication in only 1 of 22 patients, and Pugh and colleagues[33] reported 2 patients with residual posterolateral rotatory instability in his series of 40 patients. In addition, in the latter series, there were 2 radioulnar synostoses, 1 wound infection, and 4 stiff elbows requiring implant removal with release. Radiographic evidence of posttraumatic arthritis was found in 14 cases. Nonunion of the radial head fracture did not occur, but 2 fractures did exhibit delayed union.

SUMMARY

The terrible triad of the elbow is a difficult injury with historically poor outcomes. Improved experience, techniques, and implants have advanced treatment to the point where restoration of elbow stability can be expected. Careful attention to each destabilizing element of the injury pattern is essential and places high demands on the surgeon's mastery of the anatomic complexity of the elbow. Technically, the surgeon must bring every skill to bear, as soft tissue techniques, fracture repair, and joint arthroplasty are routinely required to adequately treat these complex constellations of injury.

REFERENCES

1. Morrey B. The elbow and its disorders. 2nd edition. Philadelphia: WB Saunders; 1993.
2. Mehlhoff TL, Noble PC, Bennett JB, et al. Simple dislocation of the elbow in the adult. Results after closed treatment. J Bone Joint Surg Am 1988;70: 244–9.
3. Josefsson PO, Johnell O, Gentz CF. Long-term sequelae of simple dislocation of the elbow. J Bone Joint Surg Am 1984;66:927–30.
4. Hotchkiss RN. Fractures and dislocations of the elbow. In: Rockwood CA, Green DP, Bucholz RW, et al, editors. Rockwood and Green's fractures in adults, vol. 1, 4th edition. Philadelphia: Lippincott-Raven; 1996. p. 929–1024.
5. Josefsson PO, Gentz CF, Johnell O, et al. Dislocations of the elbow and intraarticular fractures. Clin Orthop 1989;246:126–30.
6. Bryce CD, Armstrong AD. Anatomy and biomechanics of the elbow. Orthop Clin North Am 2008; 39(2):141–54.
7. Captier G, Canovas F, Mercier N, et al. Biometry of the radial head: biomechanical implications in pronation and supination. Surg Radiol Anat 2002; 24(5):295–301 [Epub 2002 Nov 1].
8. King GJ, Zarzour ZD, Patterson SD, et al. An anthropometric study of the radial head: implications in the design of a prosthesis. J Arthroplasty 2001;16(1): 112–6.
9. Halls AA, Travill A. Transmission of pressures across the elbow joint. Anat Rec 1964;150:243–7.
10. Morrey BF, An KN. Articular and ligamentous contributions to the stability of the elbow joint. Am J Sports Med 1983;11(5):315–9.
11. Josefsson PO, Gentz CF, Johnell O, et al. Surgical versus non-surgical treatment of ligamentous injuries following dislocation of the elbow joint: a prospective randomized study. J Bone Joint Surg Am 1987;69(4):605–8.
12. Closkey RF, Goode JR, Kirschenbaum D, et al. The role of the coronoid process in elbow stability; a biomechanical analysis of axial loading. J Bone Joint Surg Am 2000;82(12):1749–53.
13. Schneeberger AG, Sadowski MM, Jacob HA. Coronoid process and radial head as posterolateral

rotatory stabilizers of the elbow. J Bone Joint Surg Am 2004;86(5):975–82.
14. Weber MF, Barbosa DM, Belentani C, et al. Coronoid process of the ulna: paleopathologic and anatomic study with imaging correlation. Emphasis on the anteromedial "facet". Skeletal Radiol 2009;38(1): 61–7 [Epub 2008 Aug 15].
15. Doornberg JN, Ring D. Coronoid fracture patterns. J Hand Surg Am 2006;31(1):45–52.
16. Boone DC, Azen SP. Normal range of motion of joints in male subjects. J Bone Joint Surg Am 1979;61(5): 756–9.
17. Morrey BF, Askew LJ, Chao EY. A biomechanical study of normal functional elbow motion. J Bone Joint Surg Am 1981;63(6):872–7.
18. Morrey BF, Askey L, Chao EY. Silastic prosthetic replacement for the radial head. J Bone Joint Surg Am 1981;63:454–8.
19. Bottlang M, Madey SM, Steyers CM, et al. Assessment of elbow joint kinematics in passive motion by electromagnetic motion tracking. J Orthop Res 2000;18(2):195–202.
20. Kapandji A. Biomechanics of pronation and supination of the forearm. Hand Clin 2001;17(1):111–22.
21. O'Driscoll SW, Bell DF, Morrey BF. Posterolateral rotatory instability of the elbow. J Bone Joint Surg Am 1991;73(3):440–6.
22. Hotchkiss RN, Weiland AJ. Valgus stability of the elbow. J Orthop Res 1987;5(3):372–7.
23. Johnson JA, Beingessner DM, Gordon KD, et al. Kinematics and stability of the fractured and implant-reconstructed radial head. J Shoulder Elbow Surg 2005;14(1 Suppl S):195S–201S.
24. O'Driscoll SW, Jupiter JB, King GJ, et al. The unstable elbow. Instr Course Lect 2001;50:89–102.
25. Cohen MS, Hastings H II. Rotatory instability of the elbow: the anatomy and role of the lateral stabilizers. J Bone Joint Surg Am 1997;79(2):225–33.
26. Dunning CE, Zarzour ZD, Patterson SD, et al. Ligamentous stabilizers against posterolateral rotatory instability of the elbow. J Bone Joint Surg Am 2001;83(12):1823–8.
27. Imatani J, Ogura T, Morito Y, et al. Anatomic and histologic studies of lateral collateral ligament complex of the elbow joint. J Shoulder Elbow Surg 1999;8(6):625–7.
28. McAdams TR, Masters GW, Srivastava S. The effect of arthroscopic sectioning of the lateral ligament complex of the elbow on posterolateral rotatory stability. J Shoulder Elbow Surg 2005;14(3):298–301.
29. Olsen BS, Sojbjerg JO, Nielsen KK, et al. Posterolateral elbow joint instability: the basic kinematics. J Shoulder Elbow Surg 1998;7(1):19–29.
30. Seki A, Olsen BS, Jensen SL, et al. Functional anatomy of the lateral collateral ligament complex of the elbow: configuration of Y and its role. J Shoulder Elbow Surg 2002;11(1):53–9.

31. Sanchez-Sotelo J, Morrey BF, O'Driscoll SW. Ligamentous repair and reconstruction for posterolateral rotatory instability of the elbow. J Bone Joint Surg Br 2005;87(1):54–61.

32. Forthman C, Henket M, Ring DC. Elbow dislocation with intra-articular fracture: the results of operative treatment without repair of the medial collateral ligament. J Hand Surg Am 2007;32(8):1200–9.

33. Pugh DM, Wild LM, Schemitsch EH, et al. Standard surgical protocol to treat elbow dislocations with radial head and coronoid fractures. J Bone Joint Surg Am 2004 Jun;86-A(6):1122–30.

34. Doornberg JN, van Duijn J, Ring D. Coronoid fracture height in terrible-triad injuries. J Hand Surg Am 2006;31(5):794–7.

35. Pugh DM, McKee MD. The "terrible triad" of the elbow. Tech Hand Up Extrem Surg 2002;6(1):21–9.

36. Heim U. Surgical treatment of radial head fracture. Z Unfallchir Versicherungsmed 1992;85:3–11 [in German].

37. Gupta GG, Lucas G, Hahn DL. Biomechanical and computer analysis of radial head prostheses. J Shoulder Elbow Surg 1997;6:37–48.

38. Grewal R, MacDermid JC, Faber KJ, et al. Comminuted radial head fractures treated with a modular metallic radial head arthroplasty: study of outcomes. J Bone Joint Surg Am 2006;88(10):2192–200.

39. Moro JK, Werier J, MacDermid JC, et al. Arthroplasty with a metal radial head for unreconstructible fractures of the radial head. J Bone Joint Surg Am 2001;83:1201–11.

40. Dotzis A, Cochu G, Mabit C, et al. Comminuted fractures of the radial head treated by the Judet floating radial head prosthesis. J Bone Joint Surg Br 2006; 88(6):760–4.

41. Smets S, Govaers K, Jansen N, et al. The floating radial head prosthesis for comminuted radial head fractures: a multicentric study. Acta Orthop Belg 2000;66(4):353–8.

42. Ring D, Quintero J, Jupiter JB. Open reduction and internal fixation of fractures of the radial head. J Bone Joint Surg Am 2002;84:1811–5.

43. King GJ, Evans DC, Kellam JF. Open reduction and internal fixation of radial head fractures. J Orthop Trauma 1991;5:21–8.

44. Heim U. Combined fractures of the radius and the ulna at the elbow level in the adult. Analysis of 120 cases after more than 1 year. Rev Chir Orthop 1998;84(2):142–53 [in French].

45. Hotchkiss RN, Kasparyan NG. The medial "over the top" approach to the elbow. Tech Orthop 2000; 15(2):105–12.

46. Huh J, Krueger CA, Medvecky MJ, et al. Medial elbow exposure: over-the-top versus FCU split. Poster presented at the OTA 2011 Annual Meeting. San Antonio, TX Oct 12-15, 2011.

47. Garrigues GE, Wray WH 3rd, Lindenhovius AL, et al. Fixation of the coronoid process in elbow fracture-dislocations. J Bone Joint Surg Am 2011;93(20): 1873–81.

48. Beingessner DM, Stacpoole RA, Dunning CE, et al. The effect of suture fixation of type I coronoid fractures on the kinematics and stability of the elbow with and without medial collateral ligament repair. J Shoulder Elbow Surg 2007;16(2):213–7.

49. Calfee RP, Wilson JM, Wong AH. Variations in the anatomic relations of the posterior interosseous nerve associated with proximal forearm trauma. J Bone Joint Surg Am 2011;93(1):81–90.

50. Knight DJ, Rymaszewski LA, Amis AA, et al. Primary replacement of the fractured radial head with a metal prosthesis. J Bone Joint Surg Br 1993;75:572–6.

51. Holmenschlager F, Halm JP, Winckler S. Fresh fractures of the radial head: results with the Judet prosthesis. Rev Chir Orthop 2002;88:387–97.

52. Brinkman JM, Rahusen FT, de Vos MJ, et al. Treatment of sequelae of radial head fractures with a bipolar radial head prosthesis: good outcome after 1–4 years follow-up in 11 patients. Acta Orthop 2005;76(6):867–72.

53. Doornberg JN, Parisien R, van Duijn PJ, et al. Radial head arthroplasty with a modular metal spacer to treat acute traumatic elbow instability. J Bone Joint Surg Am 2007;89(5):1075–80.

54. Van Riet RP, Van Glabeek F, Verborgt O, et al. Capitellar erosion caused by a metal radial head prosthesis. A case report. J Bone Joint Surg Am 2004; 86:1061–4.

55. Doornberg JB, Linzel DS, Zurakowski D, et al. Reference points for radial head prosthesis size. J Hand Surg 2006;31(1):53–7.

56. Athwal GS, Rouleau DM, MacDermid JC, et al. Contralateral elbow radiographs can reliably diagnose radial head implant overlengthening. J Bone Joint Surg Am 2011;93(14):1339–46.

57. Ring D, Hannouche D, Jupiter JB. Surgical treatment of persistent dislocation or subluxation of the ulnohumeral joint after fracture-dislocation of the elbow. J Hand Surg Am 2004;29(3):470–80.

Monteggia Fractures

David Ring, MD, PhD

KEYWORDS

- Monteggia fractures • Proximal ulna • Anterior dislocation • Radial head • Radioulnar
- Radiocapitellar

KEY POINTS

- Monteggia described a fracture of the proximal third of the ulna with anterior dislocation of the radial head from both the proximal radioulnar and radiocapitellar joints.
- Application of this eponym to all injuries with radiocapitellar subluxation or dislocation has lead to some confusion.
- In addition, there are substantial differences between Monteggia injuries in children and adults.

INTRODUCTION

Monteggia described a fracture of the proximal third of the ulna with anterior dislocation of the radial head from both the proximal radioulnar and radiocapitellar joints.[1] Application of this eponym to all injuries with radiocapitellar subluxation or dislocation has led to some confusion. In addition, there are substantial differences between Monteggia injuries in children and adults.[2] With careful definition, specific subsets of patients may benefit from consideration as a separate type of Monteggia injury.

DEFINITION/CLASSIFICATION

Attempts to apply the eponym, Monteggia, to a variety of injury patterns has made the term less precise and, therefore, less useful. Monteggia injuries can be defined in 2 ways, both of which are imperfect: (1) a type of fracture-dislocation of the diaphyseal forearm with dislocation of the proximal radioulnar joint, or (2) fracture of the ulna with subluxation or dislocation of the radiocapitellar joint. The former excludes fractures at the metaphyseal or even elbow joint level that have limited proximal radioulnar joint malalignment.[3] The latter includes injuries that are types of elbow fracture-dislocations and do not involve the forearm, such as anterior olecranon fracture-dislocations.[4]

I have found it useful to consider Monteggia fractures in one of several subsets.[2,5–7] The first subset comprises diaphyseal fractures of the ulna (with or without diaphyseal fracture of the radius) and anterolateral dislocation of the radial head from the proximal radioulnar and radiocapitellar joints (Fig. 1). The second subset is made up of metaphyseal buckle fractures with anterolateral subluxation of the radiocapitellar joint, fractures that are unique to the immature skeleton (Fig. 2). The third and final group consists of the apex posterior fractures of the ulna (at the level of the diaphysis, metaphysis, or olecranon/elbow joint) with posterior dislocation of the radiocapitellar joint, with or without dislocation of the proximal radioulnar joint, and fracture of the radial head in most patients (Figs. 3 and 4).[8–10]

The traditional classification of Monteggia fractures according to direction (anterior, lateral, or posterior) was made numeric by Bado[1]: type 1, anterior; type 2, posterior; type 3, lateral; and type 4 with a concomitant radial diaphyseal fracture. It is not clear how to distinguish types 1 and 3, and type 4 seems like a subset of type 1 and 3. Therefore, I have not found Bado's classification particularly useful. The idea of Monteggia equivalents is particularly confusing and I do not recommend the use of this term or classification scheme.

Orthopaedic Hand and Upper Extremity Service, Massachusetts General Hospital, Harvard Medical School, Yawkey 2100, 55 Fruit Street, Boston, MA 02114, USA
E-mail address: dring@partners.org

Orthop Clin N Am 44 (2013) 59–66
http://dx.doi.org/10.1016/j.ocl.2012.08.007
0030-5898/13/$ – see front matter © 2013 Elsevier Inc. All rights reserved.

orthopedic.theclinics.com

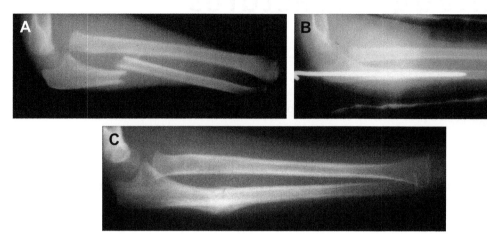

Fig. 1. A skeletally immature patient fell off playground equipment and sustained an anterolateral Monteggia injury. (*A*) Lateral radiograph shows a transverse ulna fracture in bayonet apposition and dislocation of the proximal radioulnar and radiocapitellar joints. (*B*) Open reduction and intramedullary wire fixation was performed with ancillary cast immobilization. (*C*) The fracture healed in good alignment and excellent function was obtained.

The classification of posterior Monteggia fractures proposed by Jupiter and colleagues[8] is useful primarily as way to conceptualize fracture variations that might otherwise seem disparate into a spectrum of injuries with similar management considerations. They point out that posterior Monteggia injuries are not merely forearm fracture

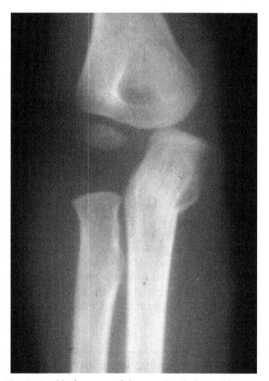

Fig. 2. Buckle fracture of the proximal ulna with anterolateral radiocapitellar subluxation in a skeletally immature patient.

dislocations but are really transitional lesions involving aspects of traumatic instability of both the elbow and the forearm. The diaphyseal posterior Monteggia fracture (type C) most resembles the classic anterolateral Monteggia fracture originally described; however, most posterior Monteggia injuries occur at the level of the metaphysis (type B) or the olecranon (type A). The final group consists of patients with complex fractures involving several levels (type D). The more proximal the fracture of the ulna lies, the greater the relative sparing of the proximal radioulnar relationship. What these fractures have in common is (1) an apex posterior fracture of the proximal ulna, (2) fracture of the radial head in most patients, and (3) avulsion of the lateral collateral ligament from the lateral epicondyle in most patients. Fractures at the level of the olecranon often include associated fracture of the coronoid.[6] All of these elements can contribute to ulnohumeral instability: apex posterior angulation of the ulna results in posterior radiocapitellar subluxation with loss of radiocapitellar contact as well as relative diminution in the effective anterior buttress of the coronoid, and fractures of the radial head and coronoid and avulsion of the LCL directly destabilize the elbow.[11,12]

EPIDEMIOLOGY

The predominant Monteggia injury in children is the anterolateral diaphyseal forearm fracture-dislocation.[7] The predominant lesion in adults is the posterior Monteggia fracture, which has been associated with osteoporosis.[2] Anterolateral diaphyseal proximal radioulnar joint fracture-dislocations are uncommonly seen in adults. The

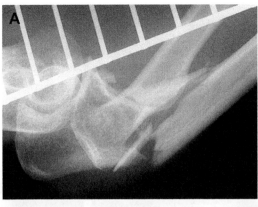

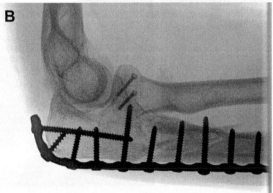

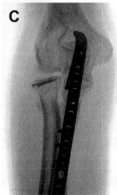

Fig. 3. Metaphyseal posterior Monteggia fracture. (*A*) Fractures at the level of the metaphysis often feature a triangular or quadrangular anterior fragment. (*B* and *C*) Contoured dorsal plate fixation can provide adequate stability to bridge this comminuted area and prevent recurrent apex posterior deformity.

anterolateral radiocapitellar subluxation and metaphyseal buckle is unique to the immature skeleton.

TREATMENT PRINCIPLES

The key treatment principle in Monteggia fractures is stable anatomic alignment of the ulna. In adults, this alignment is achieved with plate and screw fixation. Even in children, this sometimes requires open reduction and internal fixation with a plate and screws or a longitudinal wire acting as an intramedullary rod.

SPECIFIC TREATMENT TECHNIQUES
Anterolateral Fractures

Anterolateral fracture-dislocations or fracture-subluxations rarely require open reduction of the radiocapitellar/proximal radioulnar joint. Residual subluxation of these joints nearly always reflects residual malalignment of the ulna whether at the metaphyseal or diaphyseal level (**Fig. 5**).[2,6,13] In the rare situation in which exposure of the radial head is performed, it is usually sufficient to extract

the annular ligament or any other intervening structures. Restoration of the ulnar alignment is usually sufficient to stabilize the proximal radioulnar joint, provided that the interosseous ligament is intact.

In children, the ulna fracture can take one of several forms: (1) plastic deformation, (2) metaphyseal buckle, (3) greenstick (incomplete) fracture, and (4) complete displaced fractures (transverse fractures, short and long oblique fractures, and comminuted fractures). Apparent isolated proximal radioulnar dislocations usually involve some plastic deformation. Reduction of plastic deformation should be done promptly (within a few days) under general anesthesia and may require some force. Metaphyseal buckles are also reduced under anesthesia, usually require less force, and are generally stable after reduction. Green stick fractures may tend to reangulate but usually can be manipulated into a stable alignment. Complete displaced fractures can be unstable. Relatively well-aligned transverse and short oblique fractures may do well with cast treatment, but unstable displaced complete fractures merit operative treatment.

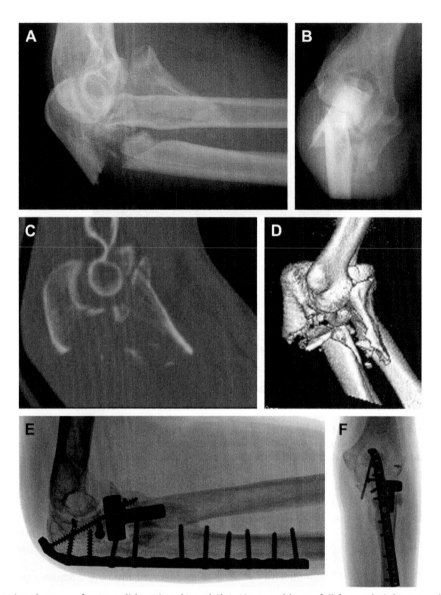

Fig. 4. Posterior olecranon fracture-dislocation. (*A* and *B*) A 40-year-old man fell from a height. Lateral and ante-roposterior radiographs after injury show an apex posterior ulna fracture, a large coronoid fracture, and poste-rior dislocation of the radial head with fracture. (*C*) Two-dimensional computed tomography is helpful but difficult to interpret. (*D*) Three-dimensional computed tomography images with and without the distal humerus are much more easily interpreted. The fractures of the coronoid and radial head are comminuted, but there is a large coronoid facet fragment to work with. (*E* and *F*) The coronoid was manipulated and reduced through the olecranon fracture; the proximal ulna was secured with a dorsal, contoured plate and screws; the radial head was replaced with a prosthesis; and the lateral collateral ligament complex was reattached to the lateral epicondyle with a suture anchor.

Reducible transverse and short oblique fractures can be stabilized with an intramedullary fixation, but long-oblique or comminuted fractures are best treated with a plate and screws. Cast immobi-lization is used for a month in children, even after operative treatment.

In adults with anterolateral displacement, stan-dard plate and screw fixation techniques with the plate applied to one of the flat surfaces of the ulna should restore forearm alignment.[6] Re-sidual radiocapitellar or proximal radioulnar subluxation usually indicate inadequate align-ment of the ulna. In fact, open reduction of the radial head should only be considered after careful reassessment of ulnar alignment and re-stored length.

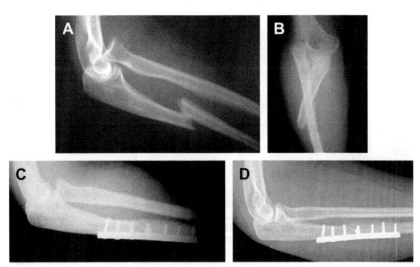

Fig. 5. Anterior (Bado I) Monteggia fracture. (*A* and *B*) The anterior Monteggia fracture (fracture of the ulnar diaphysis with anterior dislocation of the proximal radioulnar joint) is uncommon in adult patients. (*C*) Persistent subluxation of the proximal radioulnar (and radiocapitellar) joints nearly always reflects residual malalignment of the ulna. (*D*) Revision of the ulnar fixation achieved better alignment of the forearm.

Posterior Monteggia Fractures

Posterior Monteggia injuries that do not involve the ulnohumeral joint, most frequently occur at the level of the proximal ulnar metaphysis. In this location, a dorsally applied plate is preferred.[2] As previously stated, posterior Monteggia injuries with radial head fractures and lateral collateral ligament injuries demand additional attention to these destabilizing associated injuries.

When considering the posterior Monteggia injury, it is important to account for these associated characteristics because each leads to pitfalls:

1. Associated with osteoporosis—can compromise stable internal fixation.
2. Associated with LCL (Lateral collateral ligament complex) injury in about half to two-thirds of patients—can have ulnohumeral instability.
3. Many have coronoid fractures—usually large base fractures, but can also have smaller fractures similar to terrible triad injury.
4. The radial head is nearly always fractured—it is part of the posterior injury and does not make it a Bado Type 4 (radial diaphyseal fracture). The radial head fracture can compromise forearm function and elbow stability and is an important part of this injury.

Pitfalls and pearls

Pitfall: Loss of alignment or nonunion of the ulna. Pearl: Ensure anatomic reduction of the ulna fractures and use dorsal plating contoured over the olecranon process.

Take osteoporosis into account. Consider repair or replacement of the radial head fracture (**Fig. 6**).

Pitfall: Ulnohumeral instability. Pearl: If the LCL or coronoid are injured, repair them and also repair or replace the fracture of the radial head. Make sure the ulna and PRUJ/RC joint are properly aligned. If the coronoid fracture is comminuted be prepared to use a hinged external fixator temporarily (**Fig. 7**).

A midline posterior skin incision is used for all complex fractures of the proximal ulna. Traumatic wounds are incorporated. Some surgeons prefer that the incision not pass directly over the olecranon and curve it slightly.[14] A direct midline incision may cut fewer cutaneous nerves.[15]

When a plate is applied to the proximal ulna, it should be contoured to wrap around the proximal aspect of the ulna. A straight plate will only have 2 or 3 screws in metaphyseal bone proximal to the fracture. Many patients with complex proximal ulna fractures have osteopenic bone, which further compromises the strength of plate and screw fixation. Bending the plate around the proximal aspect of the olecranon provides additional screws in the proximal fragment. In addition, the most proximal screws are oriented orthogonal to the more distal screws. Finally, the most proximal screws can be long, crossing the fracture line into the distal fragment. In some cases, these screws can be directed to engage one of the cortices of the distal fragment, such as the anterior ulnar cortex.

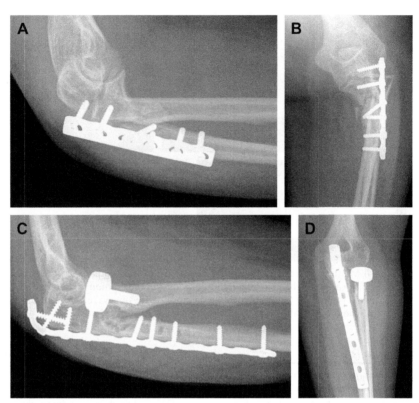

Fig. 6. Plate loosening after operative treatment of a posterior Monteggia fracture. (*A* and *B*) Posterior Monteg-gia fractures are common in older, osteoporotic patients. A plate applied to the medial or lateral surface and not contoured around the proximal ulna may have inadequate hold on the proximal metaphyseal segment. (*C* and *D*) A long dorsal contoured plate achieved healing with good alignment.

A plate applied to the dorsal surface of the proximal ulna also has several advantages over plates applied to the medial or lateral aspects of the ulna. Placing the plate along the flat dorsal surface can assist in obtaining and monitoring reduction. The dorsal surface is in the plane of the forces generated by active elbow motion so that the plate functions to a certain extent as a tension band. Finally, dorsal plate placement requires limited soft-tissue stripping.

Exposure of the ulna should preserve periosteal and muscle attachments. A plate contoured to wrap around the proximal ulna can be placed on top of the triceps insertion with few problems. This method is particularly useful when the olecranon fragment is small or fragmented. Alternatively, the triceps insertion can be incised longitudinally and partially elevated medially and laterally sufficiently to allow direct plate contact with bone.

Distally, a dorsal plate will lie directly on the apex of the ulnar diaphysis. One advantage of this situation is that the muscle need only be split sufficiently to gain access to this apex—there is no need to elevate the muscle or periosteum off either the medial or lateral flat aspect of the ulna. As an alternative to precise reduction of intervening fragmentation—once the relationship of the coronoid and olecranon facets is restored and anatomic length is re-established—the remaining fragments may be bridged, leaving their soft-tissue attachments intact. In spite of extensive fragmentation, bone grafts[16] are rarely necessary if the soft tissue attachments are preserved.[4,6]

Fractures of the radial head and coronoid process can be evaluated and often definitively treated through the exposure provided by the fracture of the olecranon process. With little additional dissection, the olecranon fragment can be mobilized proximally, providing exposure of the coronoid through the ulnohumeral joint. If the exposure of the radial head through the posterior injury is inadequate, a separate muscle interval (eg, Kocher's [between the ECU (extensor carpi ulnars) and anconeus] or Kaplan's [between the ECRL (extensor carpi radialis longus) and EDC (extensor digitorum communis)] intervals[14]) accessed by the elevation of a broad lateral skin flap can be used.

If the exposure of the coronoid is inadequate through the straight dorsal skin incision, a separate medial or lateral exposure can be developed.

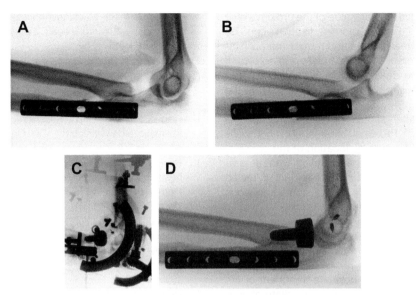

Fig. 7. Ulnohumeral instability after posterior Monteggia fracture. (*A* and *B*) Surgeons are occasionally surprised by ulnohumeral instability after what was perceived to be a forearm injury; however, posterior Monteggia injuries can include fracture of the radial head and injury to the lateral collateral ligament complex. (*C*) Open relocation of the ulnohumeral joint, restoration of radiocapitellar contact with a radial head prosthesis, repair of the lateral collateral ligament complex, and temporary hinged fixation were used to restore stability. (*D*) A stable, well-aligned elbow and forearm with good function was achieved.

Posterior olecranon fracture-dislocations often require a lateral exposure to address a fracture of the radial head or coronoid or to repair the lateral collateral ligament. When the lateral collateral ligament is injured, it is usually avulsed from the lateral epicondyle. This facilitates both exposure and repair. The lateral collateral ligament origin and common extensor musculature can be included in an anterior or posterior flap or mobilized distally.

Improved exposure of the coronoid can be obtained by releasing the origins of the radial wrist extensors from the lateral supracondylar ridge and elevating the brachialis from the anterior humerus and by excising the fractured radial head.[17,18] A medial exposure, between the 2 heads of the flexor carpi ulnaris, or by splitting the flexor-pronator mass more anteriorly, may be needed to address a complex fracture of the coronoid, particularly one that involves the anteromedial facet of the coronoid process.

The fracture of the coronoid can often be reduced directly through the elbow joint using the limited access provided by the olecranon fracture.[19–21] Provisional fixation can be obtained using Kirschner wires to attach the fragments either to the metaphyseal or diaphyseal fragments of the ulna or to the trochlea of the distal humerus when there is extensive fragmentation of the proximal ulna.[22,23] An alternative to keep in mind when there is extensive fragmentation of the proximal

ulna is the use of a skeletal distractor (a temporary external fixator).[4,22] External fixation applied between a wire driven through the olecranon fragment and up into the trochlea and a second wire in the distal ulnar diaphysis can often obtain reduction indirectly when distraction is applied between the pins. Definitive fixation can usually be obtained with screws applied under image-intensifier guidance. The screws are placed through the plate when there is extensive fragmentation of the proximal ulna. If the coronoid fracture is comminuted and cannot be securely repaired, the ulnohumeral joint should be protected with temporary hinged or static external fixation or temporary pin fixation of the ulnohumeral joint depending on the equipment and expertise available.

A long plate is contoured to wrap around the proximal olecranon. A very long plate should be considered (between 12 or 16 holes), particularly when there is extensive fragmentation of the ulnar shaft or the bone quality is poor. When the olecranon is fragmented or osteoporotic, a plate and screws alone may not provide reliable fixation. In this situation, it has proved useful to use ancillary tension wire fixation to control the olecranon fragments through the triceps insertion.

COMPLICATIONS

Plate loosening is most common in older patients when a noncontoured plate has been placed on either the medial or lateral side of the proximal ulna (see **Fig. 5**). Failed internal fixation can be salvaged with realignment and repeat internal fixation using a dorsal contoured plate and screws. If there is a bone defect or delayed union, autogenous cancellous bone graft can be applied to the fracture site.

Nonunion after simple olecranon fractures is very unusual.[24] Proximal ulnar nonunion usually occurs after a fracture-dislocation of the proximal ulna. Union can usually be achieved with restoration of anatomic length and alignment followed by contoured dorsal plate fixation and autogenous bone grafting as indicated.[24,25]

Ulnohumeral instability is sometimes a surprise to the surgeon treating a posterior Monteggia fracture. Instability is usually the result of some combination of fixation of the proximal ulna with apex dorsal deformity and inadequate treatment of the coronoid, radial head, and lateral collateral ligament complex. These often can be salvaged by secondary surgery, often including the use of hinged external fixation.[11,12,26,27]

Both the elbow and the forearm can become stiff with these injuries, particularly posterior olecranon fracture-dislocations/posterior Monteggia injuries. Proximal radioulnar synostosis occurs fairly frequently with posterior Monteggia injuries, whereas anterolateral synostosis of the elbow joint can complicate anterior Monteggia fractures.

REFERENCES

1. Bado JL. The Monteggia lesion. Clin Orthop 1967; 50:71–6.

2. Ring D, Jupiter JB, Waters PM. Monteggia fractures in children and adults. J Am Acad Orthop Surg 1998;6:215–24.

3. Bruce HE, Harvey JP, Wilson JC. Monteggia fractures. J Bone Joint Surg Am 1974;56:1563–76.

4. Ring D, Jupiter JB, Sanders RW, et al. Trans-olecranon fracture-dislocation of the elbow. J Orthop Trauma 1997;11:545–50.

5. Ring D, Jupiter JB. Fracture-dislocation of the elbow. J Bone Joint Surg Am 1998;80:566–80.

6. Ring D, Jupiter JB, Simpson NS. Monteggia fractures in adults. J Bone Joint Surg Am 1998;80: 1733–44.

7. Ring D, Waters PM. Operative fixation of Monteggia fractures in children. J Bone Joint Surg Br 1996; 78(5):734–9.

8. Jupiter JB, Leibovic SJ, Ribbans W, et al. The posterior Monteggia lesion. J Orthop Trauma 1991; 5:395–402.

9. Pavel A, Pittman JM, Lance EM, et al. The posterior Monteggia fracture. A clinical study. J Trauma 1965; 5:185–99.

10. Penrose JH. The Monteggia fracture with posterior dislocation of the radial head. J Bone Joint Surg Br 1951;33:65–73.

11. Ring D, Hannouche D, Jupiter JB. Surgical treatment of persistent dislocation or subluxation of the ulnohumeral joint after fracture-dislocation of the elbow. J Hand Surg Am 2004;29(3):470–80.

12. Ring D, Jupiter JB. Reconstruction of post-traumatic elbow instability. Clin Orthop 2000;370: 44–56.

13. Radin EL, Riseborough EJ. Fractures of the radial head. J Bone Joint Surg Am 1966;48:1055–65.

14. Morrey BF. Surgical exposures of the elbow. In: Morrey BF, editor. The elbow and its disorders. 2nd edition. Philadelphia: W B Saunders; 1993. p. 139–66.

15. Dowdy PA, Bain GI, King GJW, et al. The midline posterior elbow incision. J Bone Joint Surg Br 1995;77:696–9.

16. Ikeda M, Fukushima Y, Kobayashi Y, et al. Comminuted fractures of the olecranon. J Bone Joint Surg Br 2001;83:805–8.

17. Ring D, Jupiter JB. Operative fixation and reconstruction of the coronoid. Tech Orthop 2000; 15(2):147–54.

18. Ring D, Jupiter JB. Surgical exposure of coronoid fractures. Tech Should Elbow Surg 2002;3: 48–56.

19. Heim U. Kombinierte verletzungen von radius und ulna im proximalen unterarmsegment. Hefte Unfallchir 1994;241:61–79.

20. Heim U. Combined fractures of the upper end of the ulna and the radius in adults: a series of 120 cases. Rev Chir Orthop Reparatrice Appar Mot 1998;84: 142–53 [in French].

21. O'Driscoll SW. Technique for unstable olecranon fracture-subluxations. Oper Tech Orthop 1994;4: 49–53.

22. Mast J, Jakob RP, Ganz R. Planning and reduction techniques in fracture surgery. Heidelberg (Germany): Springer-Verlag; 1979.

23. Hastings H, Engles DR. Fixation of complex elbow fractures, part II: proximal ulna and radius fractures. Hand Clin 1997;13(4):721–35.

24. Papagelopoulos PJ, Morrey BF. Treatment of nonunion of olecranon fractures. J Bone Joint Surg Br 1994;76:627–35.

25. Ring D, Jupiter JB, Gulotta L. Atrophic nonunions of the proximal ulna. Clin Orthop 2003;409:268–74.

26. Ring D, Kloen P, Tavakolian J, et al. Loss of alignment after operative treatment of posterior Monteggia fractures: salvage with dorsal contoured plate fixation. J Hand Surg Am 2004;29:694–702.

27. McKee MD, Bowden SH, King GJ, et al. Management of recurrent, complex instability of the elbow with a hinged external fixator. J Bone Joint Surg Br 1998;80:1031–6.

Proximal Forearm Fractures

Scott G. Edwards, MD*, Jason P. Weber, MD,
Nicolai B. Baecher, MD

KEYWORDS

- Forearm fractures • Monteggia • Essex-Lopresti • Olecranon • Radial head • Terrible triad

KEY POINTS

- To prevent certain complications, surgical intervention to a traumatic elbow should be performed within 24 hours from the initial injury.
- The elbow remains an unforgiving joint, and the room for error is very small when addressing traumatic injuries to the proximal ulna and radius. Consequently, complications with elbow trauma are inevitable.
- Elbow revision surgery is one of the most difficult orthopedic surgeries in the anatomy, both conceptually and technically.

PROXIMAL FOREARM FRACTURES

Introduction

Traditionally, the discussion pertaining to elbow fractures tends to focus on supracondylar humerus fractures. Receiving less attention is the important, and arguably more complex, distal portion of the joint. This joint comprises 3 separate articulations, the ulnohumeral, radiohumeral, and radioulnar joints, each with their own goals for function and series of complications after trauma. Further, any pathology present in the elbow inevitably influences the function at the adjacent wrist either directly or indirectly. The elbow remains an unforgiving joint, and the room for error is small when addressing traumatic injuries to the proximal ulna and radius. Consequently, complications with elbow trauma are inevitable. Elbow revision surgery is one of the most difficult orthopedic surgeries in the anatomy, both conceptually and technically. This report is intended to assist surgeons in avoiding problems before they happen and managing these problems when they happen.

To prevent certain complications, surgical intervention to a traumatic elbow should be performed within 24 hours from the initial injury.[1–4] If the patient is medically unstable, delayed intervention may be elected until the patient is more stable. It is also preferable for the initial surgical intervention to be definitive and resist the temptation to return to the operating room for a staged procedure, particularly in the acute phases of the injury. Therefore, if an injury is outside the limits of the surgeon's comfort level, it is our belief that the patient's outcome would be better if the surgery was delayed until more expertise may be consulted. In other words, if given the choice of provisionally fixing the elbow or delaying surgery until definitive fixation may be obtained, the surgeon should choose the latter.

The indications for operative treatment vary depending on the particular injury. The following paragraphs summarize the indications for operative intervention for each part of the anatomy.

Indications and Contraindications

Proximal ulna

Olecranon Only completely nondisplaced olecranon fractures and comminuted fractures in elderly patients with an intact extensor mechanism may be treated nonoperatively. Any displacement of the olecranon cannot be reduced and stabilized

This manuscript was not funded.
Disclosures: JPW and NBB have nothing to disclose. SGE has a potential conflict of interest with Mylad Orthopedic Solutions.
Department of Orthopaedic Surgery, Georgetown University Hospital, 3800 Reservoir Road Northwest, Washington, DC 20007, USA
* Corresponding author. Main Building, First Floor, 3800 Reservoir Road Northwest, Washington, DC 20007.
E-mail address: sge1@gunet.georgetown.edu

Orthop Clin N Am 44 (2013) 67–80
http://dx.doi.org/10.1016/j.ocl.2012.09.001

by closed means and requires open reduction and internal fixation.

Ulnar metaphyseal/diaphyseal junction Comminuted fractures and all displaced fractures distal to the midpoint of the semilunar notch are considered unstable and require operative intervention. Although simple, nondisplaced fractures of the metaphyseal/diaphyseal junction may be treated nonoperatively, vigilance is required because these fractures suffer late displacement even with proper immobilization and patient compliance. The degree of fracture displacement in the metaphyseal/diaphyseal junction often is difficult to assess with common radiographs. Despite this challenge, it is imperative that the alignment of the proximal ulna be anatomic or the proximal radioulnar joint will be compromised.

Radial head and neck

The radial head and neck heal very well nonoperatively, making operative intervention only indicated in 3 situations: (1) open fracture, (2) bone fragments blocking supination or pronation, or (3) the buttress of the radial head is required to stabilize the elbow that otherwise has been compromised by associated ligamentous or other bony injuries. Certainly, there are parameters reported in the literature to predict joint blocking or instability, but the most reliable method to definitively determine the need for operative intervention is to take the joints through an arc of motion under local, regional, or general anesthesia. For example, local anesthesia may be administered easily in the office setting to evaluate for bony blockage. General anesthesia should be reserved for cases that are highly suspicious for instability or blockage so that the surgeon is prepared to surgically intervene in the same sitting.

Combination injuries

Combined injuries often impart complex instability patterns to the elbow and usually require operative intervention. If fracture patterns do not necessarily suggest a need for fixation by themselves, but the joint stability remains uncertain, examination under anesthesia tends to be the best way to determine the need for operative management. In these cases, general anesthesia should be used so that the surgeon is prepared to surgically intervene in the same sitting.

Management

Proximal ulna
Olecranon
Operative approach A longitudinal posterior incision is traditionally required for adequate exposure of the olecranon. The length of incision begins at the most proximal point of the olecranon, curves laterally around the olecranon prominence, and continues distally along the subcutaneous border of the ulna, enough to expose the fracture and place the necessary hardware. The subcutaneous flaps are retracted with the deep fascia and periosteum in a full-thickness manner.

Stable Transverse, displaced fractures proximal to the midpoint of the semilunar notch may be treated using several options. Traditionally tension banding techniques have been reserved for this fracture pattern. The technique was described to theoretically convert the bending forces the olecranon fragment to compressive ones. It is important to realize that this conversion of bending to compression forces has not been proven either clinically or in a biomechanics laboratory.[5] Despite this, the technique has been popular for many years. Recently, there has been a trend away from this technique for more rigid constructs, such as plating. Most would agree that plating provides a more rigid construct over tension banding.[6,7] Although it has been well accepted that tension banding has a lower profile than plating and theoretically will have less need for hardware removal, this has not been shown in the literature. Removal rates of 20%–100% have been reported for tension banding[7–10]; nearly equal to that of plating.[8,9,11] The recent application of intramedullary nailing to olecranon fractures has been proposed as a method that combines the strength of plating with the relative imperceptibility of nailing.[12] One clinical series with a minimum follow-up of 1 year showed that after implantation of a locked intramedullary nail, patients had no soft tissue irritation, and no occurrences of implant removal were reported.[13]

Fractures usually are reduced with a tenaculum under direct visualization. It is important to expose the fracture medially and laterally to assess the adequacy of reduction and remove any interposed tissue. Extending the elbow and reducing tension of the triceps tendon may facilitate reduction until provisional fixation may be placed. Once reduced, either 2 parallel 0.062-in Kirchner pins or a 7.3-mm partially threaded cancellous screw may be placed antegrade across the fracture site. Traditionally, 18-gauge stainless steel wire is used to tension the construct in a figure-8 fashion. Some surgeons have advocated using #5 braided suture for the same purpose with the intention of avoiding the soft tissue irritability of the metal wire. Whether this is successful is entirely anecdotal.

Unstable Comminuted fractures or fractures extending distal from the semilunar notch are considered unstable and are not amendable by any form f tension banding. Plating has been the standard ixation for these fractures.[14,15] Although these mplants are strong and reliable, they have high ates of soft tissue irritation and often require hardware removal.[8,9,11] One study suggests that surgeons may not be aware of the extent these mplants affect patients. In a survey distributed to 538 surgeons, most of them believed their implant removal rate to be less than 30%. Patients, however, reported a removal rate of 65%. Although surgeons believed that they removed the implant they originally placed in 92% of cases, patients reported that they only returned to the original surgeon for removal 13% of the time.[16]

Recently, intramedullary nails have been developed to overcome the shortcomings of traditional olecranon fixations in terms of soft tissue irritation and the subsequent need for removal. Of the 3 intramedullary nails currently on the market, only one (OlecraNail, Mylad Orthopedic Solutions Arlington, VA, USA) is indicated for unstable, comminuted fractures (**Fig. 1**). Similar to a locking plate, this particular nail has a fixed-angle design and rigidly stabilizes bone fragments in all planes. A recent biomechanical study compared nailing to locked plating for unstable olecranon fracture fixation in a cadaveric model.[12] Both implants controlled fragments equally well and survived an equal number of cycles. The nail, however, held fragments stable under statistically significantly greater maximal loads, suggesting that nailing may be of benefit to patients that must weight bear with their upper extremities in the immediate postoperative period. Clinically, one report showed excellent results of locked intramedullary nailing or unstable proximal ulna fracture, including comminuted fracture-dislocations and fractures involving the coronoid. All fractures achieved union by 8 weeks after surgery, and all patients had motion within 10° in the contralateral elbow within 12 weeks after surgery.[13]

Regardless of the fixation method chosen, most complications arising from unstable olecranon fracture management come from improper reduction. The sigmoid notch must be scrutinized. Anything short of a perfectly anatomic reduction will result in loss of motion in the short term and posttraumatic degeneration in the long term. One common method used by surgeons is to reduce the easily visible posterior cortex and assume that the anterior surface followed. Although this technique may work well for simple fracture patterns, one must realize that, in comminuted fracture patterns, the articular portion of the olecranon often is detached from the posterior cortex. With these fractures, the joint surface may be completely malreduced, despite an anatomic reduction of the posterior cortex (**Fig. 2**). A more appropriate technique is to reduce the bone in layers beginning with the articular surface (**Fig. 3**). Once the joint is anatomically reduced, the next layer of fragmented bone just posterior to the joint is reduced before moving on the next layer. Some fragments may be trapped between 2 other fragments, whereas others may need provisional fixation such as 0.045-in Kirchner wire. With this technique, the posterior cortex is the last layer, not the first, to be reduced. After all layers have been reduced and provisionally fixed, definitive fixation is placed, usually using one or more plates and screws or a fixed-angle intramedullary device.

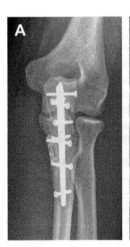
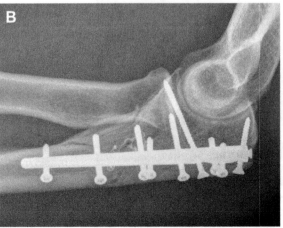

Fig. 1. Comminuted fracture-dislocation of the proximal ulna stabilized by intramedullary fixation. (*A*) Anteroposterior view; (*B*) lateral view. This implant offers the strength of a plate while being virtually imperceptible to the patient resulting in fewer soft tissue complications.

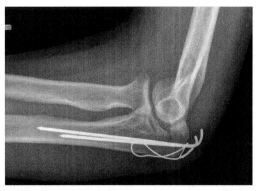

Fig. 2. Malunion of the articular surface. Approximating the posterior cortex will not assure anatomic reduction of more anterior fragments. A layered reduction technique would have been more appropriate for this patient.

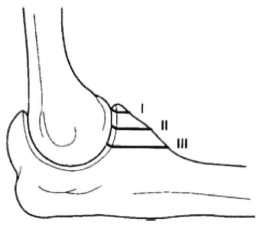

Fig. 4. Morrey classification of coronoid fractures. Type I, tip fracture. Type II, midportion fracture. Type III, base fracture.

Coronoid Management of coronoid fractures has been evolving in recent years. Only recently has the importance of its 3 dimensionality been appreciated but still not fully understood. Regan and Morrey[17] proposed a classification system based on the 2-dimensional lateral view of the elbow radiograph (**Fig. 4**). According to this familiar classification, type I (tip) fractures rarely require

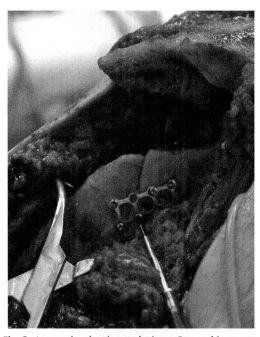

Fig. 3. Layered reduction technique. By working anterior to posterior, and distal to proximal, the surgeon is best able to reduce and provisionally stabilize fragments. Note the mini plate stabilizing the medial wall of the coronoid. The olecranon is always the last fragment to reduce.

surgical treatment, type II (midportion) fractures may require surgical treatment, and type III (base) fractures usually require surgical treatment. The coronoid can no longer be thought of as a 2-dimensional image viewed on the lateral elbow radiograph. Although fractures may appear to fragment in this fashion on plain radiographs, in actuality, coronoid fracture patterns are far more complex and often cannot be fully realized without 3-dimensional imagery.[18] Doornberg and Ring[19] found that stable anatomic fixation of the anteromedial facet of coronoid fractures was associated with better outcomes.

The coronoid may be thought of as 3 separate regions: (1) the coronoid process, (2) the medial facet, and (3) the medial wall. Each region, if compromised, may impart instability to the elbow and consequently must be addressed individually. Deforming forces generally tend to displace fragments anteriorly and distally. Fixation must resist these substantial forces, ideally, to allow early postoperative motion. Unfortunately, early motion may not be possible when dealing with these fractures. Many fixation options are tenuous and may require protection with joint immobilization. Alternatively, hinged external fixation may neutralize the deforming forces during joint motion and should be considered in select cases.

Operative approach Challenges of managing coronoid fractures reside in 3 categories: (1) identification of fracture pattern, (2) surgical approach and reduction, and (3) rigid fixation. Each category builds on the one before. As previously stated, identification of the fracture pattern and operative planning can be assisted greatly by 3-dimensional imagery techniques. Once it is determined which fragments need to be addressed, surgeons must plan their approach. This may take other associated injuries into consideration. Skin incisions tend to be irrelevant because subcutaneous tunnels may be developed readily and circumferentially around the elbow. The decision to approach the joint through facial planes seems to be more of an important issue.

We rarely use an anterior approach, however, others have used it very well. We prefer to address the coronoid from either a posterior-medial or anterior-medial approach. A posterior-medial approach is adequate for the reduction of smaller coronoid fragments or anchoring the anterior capsule back to bone. After exposing the posterior ulna, the medial portion of the ulna adjacent to the coronoid is dissected in a subperiosteal fashion. At the level of the coronoid, the ulnar nerve typically will lie in the flexor carpi ulnaris (FCU) and should be safe from a dissection remaining on the bone, but care must be exercised. Also at risk is the medical collateral ligament (MCL), which is attached to the medial facet. Detachment of the ligament should be avoided because it will compromise the vascularity of the fragment and sacrifice the stability of the joint. If reduction proves impossible without detachment of the ligament, then it should be detached at its origin on the humerus and reattached with bone tunnels or suture anchors. This proximal repair is far more predictable than reattaching distally. Reduction of the coronoid may be facilitated if there is an associated olecranon fracture. Access to the coronoid may be achieved through the window provided by a displaced olecranon fracture. After the coronoid is reduced and fixed, the olecranon may be repaired. Although this technique makes conceptual sense, its practical execution can be problematic because it is often difficult to reconfigure the semilunar notch without an intact or anatomically reduced olecranon to guide the reduction of the coronoid.

If the coronoid involvement is extensive, more exposure may be necessary. In these cases, we prefer an anterior-medial approach through the FCU.[20] It is preferable for postoperative rehabilitation to leave the posterior aspect of the FCU attached to the medial epicondyles. Once the anterior FCU is detached from the medial epicondyles and reflected distally, the exposed brachialis is retracted anteriorly for a complete view of all portions of the coronoid. We routinely decompress the ulna nerve but do not transpose. The MCL is addressed in the same manner as was previously described for the posterior-medial approach.

Once the fragments are reduced, the surgeon has an assortment of fixation techniques from which to choose. Larger fragments may be secured with screws directed either posterior to anterior or anterior to posterior depending on the particular approach. It is important to understand the limitation of screw fixation. They simply grasp the fragment rather than buttress it. Consequently, in many cases, this fixation must be protected with either temporary immobilization or neutralization with a hinged external fixator for 3 weeks. Plates may be used to buttress the deforming forces, but the amount of hardware necessary to capture all aspects of the coronoid can be substantial if multiple fragments are involved. Small fragments may be excised, and the anterior capsule may be repaired to the remaining coronoid using bone tunnels or suture anchors. Although this soft tissue repair can impart stability to the joint, it should be protected by a hinged external fixator for 3 weeks, especially if a relatively large portion of the coronoid is excised.

Garrigues and colleagues[21] examined various coronoid fixation techniques after terrible triad injuries and found that the best results were found using a suture lasso technique. This technique was more stable than repair using suture anchors or lag screws before and after repair of the lateral ulnar collateral ligament. Lag screw fixation was associated with more implant failure, and suture anchors were associated with more nonunion and malunion than the suture lasso technique.

Proximal radius

Operative approach Radial head and neck fractures may be approached through a Kocher incision. This incision may be extended proximally by detaching the extensor wad from the lateral epicondyles, but the dissection must remain anterior to the lateral collateral ligament to preserve its integrity. Should detachment be necessary, it is removed at its proximal origin on the humerus to be later reattached with suture anchors or bone tunnels. It is preferable to preserve the annular ligament. However, sacrificing the annular ligament does not lead to the instability as previous teachings have stated,[22,23] but its incision and repair will likely cause more fibrosis that may limit supination and pronation. Distal extension of the Kocher incision may be made by pronating the forearm, which displaces the posterior interosseous nerve out of the operating field. However, a recent cadaver study has shown that pronation of the forearm in a setting in which the proximal radius or radial neck is fractured does not move the posterior interosseous nerve (PIN) out of the operative field, especially if injury to the interosseous membrane is present.[24]

Simple radial head fractures may be treated with headless compression screws. A commonly displaced fragment from the anteromedial portion of the radial head, however, is not directly accessed through a lateral approach. Extreme manipulation in supination and pronation may help gain access to this problematic fragment. In some cases, screws may need to be advanced through intact bone as the displaced fragment is lagged into proper position. Overcompression of osteopenic or comminuted radial head fragments can cause the articular surface to deform and result in loss reduction. Bone grafting used in conjunction with adjustable compression screws currently on the market offer a good solution to this problem.

Plastic deformation of the radial head fragments during the time of injury may compromise reduction and overall outcome. If the radial head does not reduce easily or if it does not appear concentric with the capitellum after reduction attempts, the surgeon must suspect that some degree of plastic deformation has occurred. To remedy this problem, the articular surface must be reduced using the adjacent capitellum as a template.

This reduction will inevitably leave gaps at the base of the fragment, which should be grafted with autologous corticocancellous bone from the olecranon or bone substitute. We prefer corticocancellous grafts primarily for the adjuvant stability they provide to the fixation construct. Once the reduction is anatomic and the bone graft in place, definitive fixation is implanted.

In comminuted articular fractures that involve the radial head and neck, it is helpful to assemble the radial head on the back table. Once the articular surface has been repaired, the head can be secured to the shaft with a plate (**Fig. 5**). Alternatively, screws can be used, but we have found this to be less stable. In especially comminuted cases, rigid fixation is important because union may be delayed. The drawback to this rigid plate fixation is that it requires a significant amount of hardware to remain on the surface of the bone,

and soft tissue adhesions could pose a problem. However, Smith and colleagues[25] could not show a significant difference in elbow range of motion when comminuted radial head fractures were treated with screws alone versus plates, although there was a trend toward improved range of motion in the screws alone group. Traditionally we favor stainless steel, low-profile locking plates, given their strong screw tensile strength in providing a fixed-angle buttress and low propensity for adhesions. Recent titanium implants have improved their polishing processes, which have lessened their adhesion potential, but the tensile strength concerns still remain a question.

There has been a recent trend to replace, rather than repair or excise, radial heads.[26,27] This trend is especially true in complex fracture dislocations of the elbow[28] and has led to many reports of complications ranging from chronic pain and capitellar degeneration to rotary instability.[29,30] Improvements in design and techniques have addressed some of these complications, but surgeons should counsel patients that once a prosthetic radial is implanted, it is likely to require removal in the future. Although we prefer to repair the radial head when possible, including up to 4-part fractures, we acknowledge the short-term benefits of replacement. Radial head integrity, either comprised of bone or metal, plays an essential role in traumatic complex elbow instability. Although experts disagree on whether replacement is preferred to excision in cases of chronic radiocapitellar degeneration, most would agree that excision has no place in the acute setting, particularly if the medial collateral ligament has been compromised.[31,32] It was found that patients who underwent open reduction internal fixation for Mason type III radial head fractures have better forearm rotation and elbow extension strength along with better functional outcomes when compared with those who underwent resection

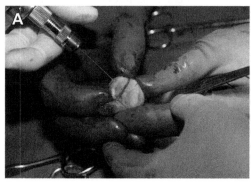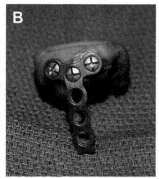

Fig. 5. Radial head reduction. (A) Assembling the radial head fragments on the back table. (B) Fully assembled radial head with plate ready to be implanted and secured to the distal portion.

of the radial head.[33] However, in isolated radial head fractures with no elbow instability, satisfactory results have been found in greater than 90% with resection of the radial head.[34]

For these cases in which the radial head is irreparable, replacement greatly helps stabilize the lateral column of the elbow and allows for early postoperative motion. Bipolar radial head prostheses for radial head fractures have been successful in 39 of 51 patients in a series, but osteolysis adjacent to the implant caused alarm when used in young or active patients.[35] Doornberg and colleagues[36] also found radiolucency adjacent to radial head implants but could not correlate this with poor outcome in short-term follow-up. These authors also recommended intentionally loosely implanting the radial head prosthesis. In addition to the use of radial head implants in the acute setting, metallic radial head arthroplasty has shown favorable results when used for chronic posttraumatic proximal forearm disorders.[37]

Our experience with partial or complete allografts has been disappointing, as resorption is common within months, which is consistent with previous reports.[38] Alternatively, we have attempted fashioning autograft iliac crest to resemble partial or complete radial heads (**Figs. 6**A and 6B). Anecdotally, incorporation of these autografts tends to be slightly more reliable, with partial grafts faring much better than complete grafts. We believe these autografts should only be considered when other options, such as prosthetic head or hinged external fixator, are not available.

Combination injuries/soft tissue injuries

Lateral collateral ligament (LCL) injuries are essentially ubiquitous in simple elbow dislocations and elbow fracture-dislcocations.[39] Fraser and colleagues[40] found that repair of the LCL with suture anchors restored the stability of the elbow in cadaveric subjects. Pollock and colleagues[41] studied 10 cadaveric elbows biomechanically with various coronoid fractures and LCL ruptures and found that in 2.5-mm anteromedial facet coronoid fractures, LCL repair restored elbow stability, whereas in 5-mm anteromedial facet coronoid fractures, stability was not restored. Pollock concluded that small anteromedial facet fractures could be treated with LCL repair alone, whereas larger types needed internal fixation. This theory is also supported by Beingessner and colleagues.[42] In a different biomechanical study done by Pollock and colleagues,[43] the elbow was stable in Morrey type II coronoid fractures as long as both collateral ligaments were intact.

Although studies have found favorable outcomes after nonoperative treatment with early range of motion for simple elbow dislocations, elbows that are unstable after simple dislocation may require repair of the collateral ligaments. Jeon and colleagues[44] repaired the MCL, LCL, or both ligaments in 13 elbows after simple dislocations that were unstable after closed reduction and found favorable results; none of the elbows redislocated. Heterotopic ossification developed in 6 of the elbows, but none of these affected the clinical outcome.

Terrible triad injuries of the elbow Frequently, injuries to the proximal forearm are not isolated to one structure. These combination injuries can be especially challenging to treat. In terrible triad injuries, where the coronoid and radial head are fractured with an elbow dislocation, results were historically poor, hence the name *terrible triad*. Treatment algorithms have been developed for treatment of this complex injury. Acutely,

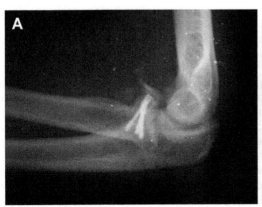 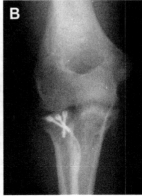

Fig. 6. Postoperative radiographs taken 3 years after reconstruction of the radial head with iliac crest autograft. (A) Lateral view; (B) anteroposterior view.

many investigators choose to (1) stabilize the coronoid fracture if it is a Morrey type II or III; (2) repair or replace the radial head; (3) repair the LCL and assess for stability; (4) if unstable, then repair the MCL and again assess stability; and (5) if still unstable, consider dynamic external fixation.[45] Some investigators skip step 4 and place an external fixator if the elbow is unstable after repair of the LCL.[46] However, some surgeons repair the MCL after treatment of the radial head, coronoid, and LCL in terrible triad injuries even if the elbow is thought to be stable after repair of the LCL.[47,48]

The LCL is always torn in terrible triad injuries and should be repaired with suture anchors or intraosseous sutures. Suture anchors and intraosseous sutures have equal failure loads when repairing the MCL, and both have higher failure loads when they are pretensioned.[49] Forthman and colleagues[50] examined 34 patients with intra-articular fracture dislocations of the elbow. Thirty of these patients had terrible triad injuries. Forthman and colleagues[50] (1) treated the coronoid fracture (most frequently with intraosseous sutures), (2) repaired or replaced the radial head, and (3) repaired the LCL. All elbows were considered stable, and the MCL was not repaired. Elbow instability developed in 2 of the patients because of noncompliance, whereas 25 of the remaining 32 patients experienced good or excellent results. Lindenhovius and colleagues[51] treated terrible triad injuries in a similar manner as Forthman and colleagues,[50] although 3 patients in his study were placed in a dynamic external fixator and also showed favorable outcomes. In addition, the Lindenhovius study noted an improved flexion arc in patients treated within 2 weeks of injury versus patients treated more than 3 weeks from the injury.

MONTEGGIA FRACTURES

A significant amount of energy is required to fracture the bones of the forearm. Most injuries are sustained from falls, motor vehicle accidents, or a direct blow. A not-uncommon cause of forearm trauma is gunshot wounds. Often, significant injuries may be sustained to the muscles, tendons, and nerves of the forearm; this can potentially carry the risk of significant disability and difficulty recovering from and adapting to the injuries.

In any injury pattern that could or may have imparted trauma to both radial and ulnar sided structures it is important to assess the interosseous membrane. Examples of such injuries are Monteggia and Monteggia-equivalent injuries and radial head fractures.

Monteggia fractures are more accurately categorized as fracture-dislocations of the proximal forearm. These injuries are characterized by a dislocation of the radial head occurring with a fracture of the proximal third of the ulna. The concept of a spectrum of Monteggia-type injuries was the contribution of Bado in 1967.[52] Looking at posterior Monteggia lesions and ulnar fracture patterns, Jupiter and colleagues[53] further refined the classification in 1991. Compared with all forearm fractures, Monteggia-type injuries are uncommon, comprising about 5% of all such injuries. Giovanni Monteggia first described the classic pattern in 1814, describing an injury consisting of an anterior dislocation of the radial head combined with a fracture of the proximal third of the ulna.[54] Bado type I injuries seem to be the most common in adults, comprising about 60%–80% of cases. Type II injuries occur around 15%–30% of the time.[55]

Mechanism of Injury

It is not clearly understood how these injuries are sustained. Proposed mechanisms include a direct blow to the elbow, fall on an outstretched arm, and a possible role of biceps as a violent anterior force on the proximal radius. The position of the hand when the injury occurs is thought to influence whether the injury is anterior or posterior. Anterior Monteggia injuries are thought to occur with the hand in a hyperpronated position, thus imparting a levering force on the proximal radius leading to anterior dislocations. Posterior type injuries have been thought to occur with the hand in a hypersupinated position, thus tightening many of the soft tissue constraints of the elbow and encouraging the radial head to dislocate posteriorly. Lateral injuries may be associated with a direct blow to the medial aspect of the elbow causing sufficient varus moment to dislocate the head laterally.

Preoperative history and considerations

Most patients will complain of pain around the elbow and a block to full motion of the elbow, specifically, difficulty with elbow flexion and forearm rotation. Injury to the PIN is not uncommon, occurring in about 17% of all Monteggia-type injuries. Most of these injuries are of a neuropraxic nature. The etiology of PIN injury is thought to be stretching of the nerve as it carried with the radial head as it dislocates. Other nerves of the forearm such as the anterior interosseous nerve, the median nerve, and the ulnar nerve have been noted to be injured on occasion with this injury type. Like radial nerve palsies in the setting of a humeral shaft fracture, PIN palsy is not an indication to acutely explore the nerve. Most PIN palsies will return with time. Surgical exploration of the nerve should be considered starting at 8 weeks if there has been no improvement or return of PIN function by that time.

Diagnostic imaging should include anteroposterior and lateral x-rays of the elbow, forearm, and wrist to ensure a full understanding of the affected anatomy. Oblique views may help if the exact injury pattern, especially around the elbow and wrist, is unclear. It is unusual that advanced imaging (eg, computed tomography or magnetic resonance imaging [MRI]) is necessary to define the injury. As in many other fracture patterns, high-energy injuries will typically be marked by more comminution and segmental fracture patterns.

Important aspects to note on plain radiographs include radial head reduction as well as coronoid and olecranon integrity. The relationship between the radial shaft, head, and capitellum is a key point. When imaging a properly reduced radial head from any projection, it should be possible to draw a straight line through the center of the capitellum, the center of the radial head, and on through the radial shaft. It is possible for the radial head to either spontaneously reduce or be reduced before the obtainment of plain films. Therefore, suspicion of radial head dislocation should still be considered even in the setting of a radiologically reduced head. Together, the coronoid process and olecranon provide most of the boney congruency of the elbow joint. These 2 structures should be inspected carefully on plain film to rule out any fractures.

Classification Bado classification includes the following:

- Type I (~60%)—Anterior radial head dislocation with an apex anterior proximal ulna fracture
- Type II (~15%)—Posterior radial head dislocation with an apex posterior proximal ulna fracture
- Type III—Lateral radial head dislocation with a proximal ulna fracture (typically in the metaphyseal region)
- Type IV—Anterior radial head dislocation with both a proximal radial fracture and a proximal ulna fracture

Jupiter classification of Bado type II injuries includes the following:

- Type IIA—Ulna fracture located at the level of the trochlear notch
- Type IIB—Ulna fracture located at the level of the metadiaphyseal junction

- Type IIC—Ulna fracture located in the diaphysis
- Type IID—Ulna fracture extends into the proximal diaphysis

Management of Monteggia fractures

In adults, the current standard is for all Monteggia fractures and equivalent injuries to be treated with open reduction and internal fixation. The radial head may often be reduced in a closed fashion after the ulna is reduced anatomically. Difficulty reducing the radial head may either indicate an error in the reduction of the ulna (nonanatomic) or the presence of interposed tissue laterally. If this is the case, the radial head may need to be reduced in an open fashion through a separate lateral incision. The block to reduction may be the PIN, hence, the importance of opening the lateral elbow joint when the radial head proves irreducible by closed means.

As in many other scenarios, timing of surgery largely depends on the condition of the soft tissue envelope around the elbow.

All injuries should be well appreciated through the preoperative physical examination and all necessary imaging studies. These will include orthogonal plain films and may include computed tomography scans with or without 3-dimensional reconstructions, and even MRI in some cases.

The patient will typically be placed in either a lateral decubitus position (most commonly) or supine position with the arm placed across the chest. Using a bump (either rolled towels or a bag of saline) to elevate the ipsilateral shoulder can be beneficial to maintaining the arm across the chest.

Surgical approach

The standard approach to Monteggia injuries is to make a midline posterior skin incision. This incision should be lateral to the prominence of the olecranon. This is essentially the same approach used to address isolated olecranon or proximal ulna fractures. The interval between the flexor carpi ulnaris and anconeus is used to carry the dissection deeper; this is an internervous plane. By releasing the anconeus off its insertion in the proximal ulna, the radial head can be accessed if it needs to be addressed (the Boyd approach).[56] This technique is only possible before the ulnar fracture has been addressed. The access the ulna fracture provides is needed to appropriately visualize the radial head via this approach. Alternatively, a separate lateral incision can be made to address the radial head.

Although radial head reduction is usually accomplished after fixation of the ulnar injuries, radial head fixation should be addressed before fixing the ulna. However, if the injury is too comminuted to be repaired, and a radial head replacement is being contemplated, this technique ought to be performed after reduction and fixation of the ulna, because a proper humeral-ulnar relationship is needed to properly size the radial head implant.

Fixation of the ulna will depend on the location of the fracture. Fractures that do not involve the olecranon's articular surface can either be plated laterally (in an attempt to avoid hardware prominence) or subcutaneously in a more traditional fashion.

As a general rule, fixation of the ulna when it extends into the articular surface will proceed from distal to proximal. The goal, as in any intra-articular fracture, is anatomic reduction of the articular surface. Fragments may be fixed using interfragmentary screw or Kirschner wires. Kirschner wires can be of particular advantage in provisionally holding fragment fixation before definitive fixation with a dorsally placed plate. Alternatively, if the fracture pattern allows, larger fragments can be fixed with lag screw techniques. Coronoid fractures are often accessible via existing fracture lines in the olecranon. If a coronoid fracture is present but cannot be visualized adequately, an olecranon osteotomy may be performed to provide increased access to the articular surface. Because of the triceps insertion, the most proximal olecranon fragment will be the last to be attached to the reconstructed ulna.

Beingessner and colleagues[57] reported on 16 patients with Bado type IID injuries and had satisfactory outcomes. They addressed the order of fixation as follows: (1) repair or replacement of the radial head; (2) reduction of the ulnar shaft, including the anterior oblique cortical fragment (if present); (3) reduction and stabilization of the coronoid process with either screws or transosseous sutures; (4) reduction and fixation of the olecranon process to the ulnar shaft and definitive fixation of the ulnar shaft component of the injury; (5) repair of osseous ulnar insertion of the medial collateral ligament or lateral collateral ligament; and (6) repair of the humeral origin of the lateral ulnar collateral ligament.

Complications in the treatment of the Monteggia fractures

Monteggia fractures are difficult injuries to treat. As fracture-dislocations, the extent and diversity of tissue injured is extensive, and the elbow is an unforgiving joint to begin with, especially considering the complexity of the articular surface, and the combination of rotational motion through the radiocapitellar articulation and flexion-extension through the humeral-ulnar articulation. One multi center study from Belgium found a 43% overall complication rate in the treatment of Monteggia fractures, with 46% of the patients reporting unsatisfactory outcomes.

Common complications in the treatment of these injuries are posterior interosseous nerve palsies, redislocation or subluxation, synostosis and loss of motion.

Nerve injury Neuropraxia of the posterior interosseous nerve is common in these injuries. The injury can occur from traction of the nerve with either lateral or anterior displacement of the proximal radius, entrapment at the arcade of Frosche or from direct trauma (usually blunt) to the nerve Most cases spontaneously resolve, and, as mentioned earlier, there is little reason to explore the PIN acutely.

Subluxation Failure to properly reconstruct the ulna in an anatomic position frequently can lead to repeated dislocation or subluxation of the radial head because of the incongruity at the articular surfaces. Apex dorsal ulnar fractures may have unrecognized comminution through the volar cortex that is not appreciated at the time of fixation. This can result in residual apex dorsal angulation leading to recurrent subluxation or dislocation of the radial head. Malunion may also occur through inadequate plate strength. Semitubular and pelvic reconstruction plates are not generally strong enough to resist the forces across the proximal ulna and, in our experience, may frequently experience bending through the plate and subsequent angular malunions.

Synostosis Synostosis is a feared complication of this injury, with potentially devastating implications for forearm rotation. Factors that seem to increase the change of postoperative synostosis are high-energy injuries, fractures of the radius and ulna at the same level, and use of the Boyd approach to radial head.

The following factors have been associated with worse outcomes: type II injuries, Jupiter type IIA injuries, fractures involving the radial head, coronoid fractures, and complications that require further surgical treatment for resolution.[55]

ESSEX-LOPRESTI INJURIES
Introduction

A rare variation in forearm fracture patterns is the Essex-Lopresti injury. This is a complex traumatic injury to the interosseous membrane of the forearm resulting in a loss of the normal radio-ulnar stability. It was first described by Essex-Lopresti in 1951.[58] It is thought to occur primarily after a fall onto an outstretched hand. The force is transmitted proximally through the interosseous membrane to the radial head. The resulting injury is typically noted by a fracture of the radial head and disruption of the interosseous membrane and distal radial-ulnar joint.

Preoperative history and considerations

It is an easy and frequent clinical mistake to overlook an Essex-Lopresti injury. Patients typically complain of primary of elbow pain and may be distracted from noticing a painful injury in the distal forearm. Often, imaging may only include the elbow, and the radial head may distract the examining physicians from taking a close look at the distal forearm. Full radiographs of the entire forearm should be obtained in the setting of a radial head fracture to help rule out concomitant injuries, proving the old adage of imaging the joint above and below the injury.

To evaluate the interosseous membrane, a careful physical examination is required. Given the painful nature of these injuries, sedation or adequate analgesia may be required to obtain a sufficient examination. The surgeon should assess the integrity of the membrane by attempting to translate the radius proximally in a longitudinal fashion. If more than 3 mm of translation is noted, this indicates injury to the interosseous membrane. More than 6 mm of translation is suspicious for injury to both the interosseous membrane and the triangular fibrocartilage complex.

Diagnostic imaging can supplement the physical examination. Plain radiographs are the standard initial imaging modality. With an Essex-Lopresti injury, widening may be seen at the distal radioulnar joint (DRUJ) or shortening of the radius in relation to the distal ulna (giving the appearance of positive ulnar variance). MRI and ultrasound scan are the most useful modalities for directly assessing a suspected interosseous injury, because they may reveal injury to the relevant soft tissue structures in question.[59] Based on x-ray imaging, Edwards and Jupiter[60] published a classification of Essex-Lopresti injuries in 1988 centered around the nature of the accompanying radial head fracture.

Classification

Edwards-Jupiter Classification of Essex-Lopresti Injuries

- Type 1—Large displaced radial head fractures
- Type 2—Severely comminuted radial head fractures
- Type 3—Chronic radial fractures with irreducible radial migration

Management

Commonly, the only treatment for an Essex-Lopresti injury is repair or replacement of the radial head. In the acute setting, after treatment of the radial head, the forearm should be examined for longitudinal stability. If instability is found, then the forearm can be immobilized in supination using a splint and then cast, Kirschner wires, or 3.5-mm screws. More recently, support for reconstruction of the central band of the interosseous membrane (IOM) has surfaced in the acute setting. However, this evidence is only seen in studies of cadaveric subjects. Most surgeons do not reconstruct the IOM in an acute Essex-Lopresti injury. However,

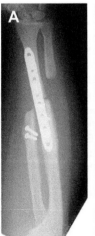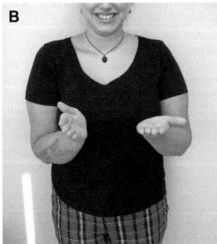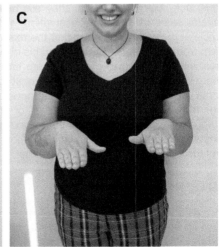

Fig. 7. One-bone forearm conversion. (*A*) Radiograph; (*B*) supination; (*C*) pronation. Note the short arc of rotation moving through the radiocarpal and midcarpal joints.

even with an intact radial read, the central band of the IOM provides 71% of the longitudinal stability of the forearm.[61] Studies of cadaveric subjects have found that replacing the radial head alone while ignoring the IOM injury does not completely restore longitudinal stability to the forearm.[62,63] Reconstruction of the central band of the IOM using nylon, palmaris longus tendon, flexor carpi radialis tendon, bone patellar tendon bone, suture button construct, pronator teres, Achilles tendon allograft, and AC Graft Rope (Arthrex, Naples, FL) have all been described.[64] There are no clinical studies treating acute Essex-Lopresti injuries with IOM reconstruction. Ultimate salvage for this injury is a one-bone forearm conversion, but it is not a "death sentence" as most patients are reasonably pleased with the short arc of supination and pronation provided through the radiocarpal and midcarpal joints (See **Fig. 7**).

SUMMARY

The only thing more challenging than repairing a traumatized proximal forearm is to revise what had failed. A large portion of this article focuses on aspects of the management of acute trauma because prevention of complications cannot be overemphasized. Despite adhering to the dogma presented here, outcomes can be unpredictable in the proximal forearm. Revision elbow surgery is almost the norm rather than the exception. Unfortunately, the literature has little guidance for revision surgery. The literature describes well that problems of the proximal ulna and radius exist but fails to clearly indicate what to do when these problems occur. This article attempts to supplement what is known in the literature with the author's anecdotal experience. Although some of the recommendations lack scientific support, they are based on several years of trial and observation. With this article, it is the author's hope that the reader may learn from his or her successes and his or her failures without having to discover them first hand. There is good reason for a wave of angst to overcome surgeons first gazing at radiographs depicting traumatized a proximal ulna or radius. Surgeons know that there will be a good chance they will be seeing these patients for a long time, and the journey will not be easy for either.

REFERENCES

1. O'Driscoll S. Optimizing stability in distal humeral fracture fixation. J Shoulder Elbow Surg 2005; 14(1 Suppl S):186S–94S.
2. Sanchez-Sotelo J, Torchia M, O'Driscoll S. Complex distal humeral fractures: internal fixation with a principle-based parallel-plate technique. Surgical technique. J Bone Joint Surg Am 2008; 90(Suppl 2 Pt 1):31–46.
3. Plancher KD, Lucas TS. Fracture dislocations of the elbow in athletes. Clin Sports Med 2001;20(1): 59–76.
4. Constant C. Injuries to the elbow. J R Coll Surg Edinb 1990;35(Suppl 6):S31–2.
5. Hutcinson D, Horwitz D, Ha G, et al. Cyclic loading of olecranon fracture fixation constructs. J Bone Joint Surg Am 2003;85-A(5):831–7.
6. Newman S, Mauffrey C, Krikler S. Olecranon fractures. Injury 2009;40(6):575–81.
7. Hume MC, Wiss DA. Olecranon fractures. A clinical and radiographic comparison of tension band wiring and plate fixation. Clin Orthop Relat Res 1992;(285): 229–35.
8. Lindenhovius A, Brouwer K, Doornberg J, et al. Long-term outcome of operatively treated fracture dislocations of the olecranon. J Orthop Trauma 2008;22(5):325–31.
9. Rommens P, Küchle R, Schneider R, et al. Olecranon fractures in adults: factors influencing outcome. Injury 2004;35(11):1149–57.
10. Macko D, Szabo R. Complications of tension-band wiring of olecranon fractures. J Bone Joint Surg Am 1985;67(9):1396–401.
11. Bailey CS, MacDermid J, Patterson SD, et al. Outcomes of plate fixation of olecranon fractures. J Orthop Trauma 2001;15(8):542–8.
12. Klimkiewicz J, Argintar E, Martin B, et al. Nail vs plate biomechanical comparison in unstable olecranon fractures. Poster presentation. Annual Meeting American Society for Surgery of the Hand. San Francisco, October 3–5, 2009.
13. Argintar E, Cohen MS, Eglseder WA, et al. Clinical results of olecranon fractures treated with multiplanar locked intramedullary nailing. J Orthop Trauma 2012. [Epub ahead of print].
14. Buijze G, Kloen P. Clinical evaluation of locking compression plate fixation for comminuted olecranon fractures. J Bone Joint Surg Am 2009;91(10):2416–20.
15. Sahajpal D, Wright TW. Proximal ulna fractures. J Hand Surg Am 2009;34(2):357–62.
16. Edwards SG, Cohen MS, Lattanza LL, et al. Surgeon perceptions and patient outcomes regarding proximal ulna fixation: a multicenter experience. J Shoulder Elbow Surg 2012. [Epub ahead of print].
17. Regan W, Morrey B. Classification and treatment of coronoid process fractures. Orthopedics 1992;15(7): 845–8.
18. O'Driscoll S, Jupiter J, Cohen M, et al. Difficult elbow fractures: pearls and pitfalls. Instr Course Lect 2003; 52:113–34.
19. Doornberg J, Ring D. Fracture of the anteromedial facet of the coronoid process. J Bone Joint Surg Am 2006;88A(10):2216–24.

20. Kasparyan NG, Hotchkiss RN. Dynamic skeletal fixation in the upper extremity. Hand Clin 1997;13: 643–63.

21. Garrigues G, Wray W, Lindenhovius A, et al. Fixation of the coronoid process in elbow fracture-dislocations. J Bone Joint Surg Am 2011;93:1873–81.

22. Bhaskar A. Missed Monteggia fracture in children: is annular ligament reconstruction always required? Indian J Orthop 2009;43(4):389–95.

23. Cohen M, Hastings H. Rotatory instability of the elbow. The anatomy and role of the lateral stabilizers. J Bone Joint Surg Am 1997;79(2):225–33.

24. Calfee R, Wilson J, Wong A. Variations in the anatomic relations of the posterior interosseous nerve with proximal forearm trauma. J Bone Joint Surg Am 2011;93:81–90.

25. Smith AM, Morrey BF, Steinmann SP. Low profile fixation of radial head and neck fractures: surgical technique and clinical experience. J Orthop Trauma 2007;21:718–24.

26. Ring D, Quintero J, Jupiter J. Open reduction and internal fixation of fractures of the radial head. J Bone Joint Surg Am 2002;84-A(10):1811–5.

27. Ring D, King D. Radial head arthroplasty with a modular metal spacer to treat acute traumatic elbow instability. J Bone Joint Surg Am 2007;89: 1075–80.

28. Ring D, Jupiter JB, Zilberfarb J. Posterior dislocation of the elbow with fractures of the radial head and coronoid. J Bone Joint Surg Am 2002;84A:547–51.

29. Calfee R, Madom I, Weiss A. Radial head arthroplasty. J Hand Surg Am 2006;31(2):314–21.

30. Birkedal J, Deal D, Ruch D. Loss of flexion after radial head replacement. J Shoulder Elbow Surg 2004;13(2):208–13.

31. Pike J, Athwal G, Faber K, et al. Radial head fractures—an update. J Hand Surg Am 2009;34(3): 557–65.

32. Rosenblatt Y, Athwal G, Faber K. Current recommendations for the treatment of radial head fractures. Orthop Clin North Am 2008;39(2):173–85.

33. Ikeda M, Sugiyama K, Kang C, et al. Comminuted fractures of the radial head: comparison of resection and internal fixation. J Bone Joint Surg Am 2005; 87A:76–84.

34. Antuna S, Sanchez-Marquez J, Barco R. Long-term results of radial head resection following isolated radial head fractures in patients younger than forty years old. J Bone Joint Surg Am 2010;92:558–66.

35. Popovic N, Lemaire R, Georis P, et al. Midterm results with bipolar radial head prosthesis: radiographic evidence of loosening at the bone-cement interface. J Bone Joint Surg Am 2007;89:2469–76.

36. Doornberg J, Parisien R, van Duijn J, et al. Radial head arthroplasty with modular metal spacer to treat acute traumatic elbow instability. J Bone Joint Surg Am 2007;89:1075–80.

37. Shore BJ, Mozzon JB, MacDermid JC, et al. Chronic posttraumatic elbow disorders treated with metallic radial head arthroplasty. J Bone Joint Surg Am 2008;90A:271–80.

38. Karlstad R, Morrey B, Cooney W. Failure of fresh-frozen radial head allografts in the treatment of Essex-Lopresti injury. A report of four cases. J Bone Joint Surg Am 2005;87(8):1828–33.

39. McKee MD, Schemitsch EH, Sala MJ, et al. The pathoanatomy of lateral ligamentous disruption in complex elbow instability. J Shoulder Elbow Surg 2003;12:391–6.

40. Fraser GS, Pichora JE, Ferreira LM, et al. Lateral collateral ligament repair restores initial varus stability of the elbow: an in vitro biomechanical study. J Orthop Trauma 2008;22:615–23.

41. Pollock JW, Brownhill J, Ferriera L, et al. The effect of anteromedial facet fractures of the coronoid and lateral collateral ligament injury on elbow stability and kinematics. J Bone Joint Surg Am 2009;91: 1448–58.

42. Beingessner DM, Stacpoole RA, Dunning CE, et al. The effect of suture fixation of type I coronoid fractures on the kinematics and stability of the elbow with and without medial collateral ligament repair. J Shoulder Elbow Surg 2007;16:213–7.

43. Pollock JW, Pichora J, Brownhill J, et al. The influence of type II coronoid fractures, collateral ligament injuries, and surgical repair on the kinematics and stability of the elbow: an in vitro biomechanical study. J Shoulder Elbow Surg 2009;18:408–17.

44. Jeon IH, Kim SY, Kim PT. Primary ligament repair for elbow dislocation. Keio J Med 2008;57:99–104.

45. Pugh DM, Wild LM, Schemitsch EH, et al. Standard surgical protocol to treat elbow dislocations with radial head and coronoid fractures. J Bone Joint Surg Am 2004;86A:1122–30.

46. Egol KA, Immerman I, Paksima N, et al. Fracture-dislocation of the elbow functional outcome following treatment with a standardized protocol. Bull NYU Hosp Jt Dis 2007;65:263–70.

47. Jeong WK, Oh JK, Hwang JH, et al. Results of terrible triads of the elbow: the advantage of primary restoration of medial structure. J Orthop Sci 2010; 15:612–9.

48. Zeiders GJ, Patel MK. Management of unstable elbows following complex fracture-dislocations—the "terrible triad" injury. J Bone Joint Surg Am 2008;90:75–84.

49. Pichora JE, Furukawa K, Ferreira LM, et al. Initial repair strengths of two methods for acute medial collateral ligament injuries of the elbow. J Orthop Res 2007;25:612–6.

50. Forthman C, Henket M, Ring DC. Elbow dislocation with intraarticular fracture: the results of operative treatment without repair of the medial collateral ligament. J Hand Surg Am 2007;32:1200–9.

51. Lindenhovius AL, Jupiter JB, Ring D. Comparison of acute versus subacute treatment of terrible triad injuries of the elbow. J Hand Surg Am 2008;33:920–6.

52. Bado J. The Monteggia lesion. Clin Orthop Relat Res 1967;50:71.

53. Jupiter JB, Leibovic SJ, Ribbans W, et al. The posterior Monteggia lesion. J Orthop Trauma 1991;5:395–402.

54. Monteggia GB. Instituzioni chirurgiche. 2nd edition. Milan (Italy): G. Masperp; 1813–1815.

55. Konrad GG, Kundel K, Kreuz PC, et al. Monteggia fractures in adults: long-term results and prognostic actors. J Bone Joint Surg Br 2007;89B:354–60.

56. Speed J, Boyd H. Treatment of fractures of the ulna with dislocation of the head of the radius (Monteggia fracture). JAMA 1940;115:1699–705.

57. Beingessner DM, Nork SE, Agel J, et al. A fragment-specific approach to type IID Monteggia elbow fracture-dislocations. J Orthop Trauma 2011;25:414–9.

58. Essex-Lopresti PJ. Fractures of the radial head with distal radio-ulnar dislocation; report of two cases. Bone Joint Surg Br 1951;33B(2):244–7.

59. Rodriguez-Martin J, Pretell-Mazzini J. The role of ultrasound and magnetic resonance imaging in the evaluation of the forearm interosseous membrane. Skeletal Radiol 2011;40(12):1515–22.

60. Edwards GS Jr, Jupiter JB. Radial head fractures with acute distal radioulnar dislocation. Essex-Lopresti revisited. Clin Orthop Relat Res 1988;234:61–9.

61. Hotchkiss RN, An KN, Sowa DT, et al. An anatomic and mechanical study of the interosseous membrane of the forearm: pathomechanics of proximal migration of the radius. J Hand Surg 1989;14A:256–61.

62. Tomaino MM, Pfaeffle J, Stabile K, et al. Reconstruction of the interosseous ligament of the forearm reduces load on the radial head in cadavers. J Hand Surg 2003;28B:267–70.

63. Birkbeck DP, Failla JM, Hoshaw SJ, et al. The interosseous membrane affects load distribution in the forearm. J Hand Surg 1997;22A:975–80.

64. Drake ML, Farber GL, White KL, et al. Restoration of longitudinal forearm stability using a suture button contruct. J Hand Surg 2010;35A:1981–5.

Complex Distal Radius Fractures

Stephen A. Kennedy, MD, FRCSC[a], Douglas P. Hanel, MD[b],*

KEYWORDS

- Distal radius • Fracture • Wrist • Trauma • Complex • Intra-articular • Open

KEY POINTS

- Complex distal radius fractures are high-energy injuries of the wrist with articular disruption, ligamentous instability, significant comminution, soft tissue injury, and/or neurovascular impairment.
- The comprehensive management of these injuries requires a thorough understanding of wrist functional anatomy and familiarity with a wide selection of approaches and fixation options.
- Outcome is determined by multiple factors and depends greatly on the soft tissue injury, patient factors, and management and the adequacy of restoration of osseous and ligamentous relationships.

Distal radius fractures are the most common fractures seen in emergency departments.[1] Most are low-energy injuries that are managed well with closed reduction and immobilization or splinting and outpatient surgery. Complex distal radius fractures, however, are high-energy injuries that may have severe articular disruption, high degrees of comminution, and/or ligamentous instability. They are associated with soft tissue injury, neurologic or vascular impairment, and require greater urgency and resources. Treatment may be further complicated by the need to address multiple injuries.

Myriad treatment options exist for complex distal radius fractures, with various surgical approaches, reduction techniques, fixation options, and reconstructive procedures available. However, there are important core principles upon which to guide treatment. This article reviews an approach that involves structured evaluation, aggressive soft tissue management, early reduction and skeletal stabilization, and a columnar approach to definitive care of the osseous and ligamentous injuries.[2,3]

EVALUATION AND INITIAL MANAGEMENT

The assessment of complex distal radius fractures requires an organized approach to assess injury severity and identify associated injuries. The location and severity of pain, and history of neurologic or vascular symptoms help identify arterial injury, nerve injury, or compartment syndrome. The timing of neurologic symptoms may indicate whether there is ongoing or progressive nerve compression (**Box 1**).[4]

Physical examination is the mainstay of assessment of complex distal radius injuries. The entire limb is closely examined to evaluate soft tissue integrity, degree of deformity, instability, tenderness, and neurovascular status. Pain and

No funding support was provided for this work.
Douglas Hanel is a consultant for Aptis Medical LLC.
Stephen Kennedy has no financial relationships to disclose.
[a] Hand and Microvascular Surgery, Department of Orthopaedics and Sports Medicine, University of Washington–Roosevelt II, 4245 Roosevelt Way Northeast, Box 354740, Seattle, WA 98105, USA; [b] Department of Orthopaedics and Sports Medicine, Harborview Medical Center, University of Washington, 325 Ninth Avenue, Box 303490, Seattle, WA 98104, USA
* Corresponding author.
E-mail address: dhanel@u.washington.edu

Management of airway, ventilation, and circulation precedes evaluation of the limb.

Focused history of pain and neurovascular symptoms can identify urgent syndromes such as nerve compression, arterial insufficiency, or compartment syndrome.

Assessment and documentation of soft tissue status and neurovascular compromise are essential. Objective documentation assists in identifying progression of neurovascular deficits.

Tourniquets should be avoided for control of bleeding from open wounds, as they prevent perfusion of already compromised tissues. Pressure dressings are adequate.

Ensure that gross deformities are realigned if necessary; wounds are irrigated of gross contamination and dressed; and analgesics, antibiotics, and tetanus prophylaxis are administered as appropriate.

Initial standardized radiographs that include postero-anterior, lateral, and oblique views of the wrist can provide a wealth of information. Traction and reduction views under fluoroscopy provide further information about specific fragments and instability patterns.

After reduction, lateral 10-degree oblique views may better visualize the lunate facet.

Computed tomography (CT) scan may be performed if there are specific concerns such as dye punch fracture. This is dependent on surgeon preference and resource availability, and may be done after debridement and application of a radiolucent external fixator.

tenderness will limit some aspects of evaluation. Perfusion is assessed with color, warmth, pulse oximetry, and/or Doppler ultrasound as needed. Neurologic examination is documented with graded motor strength and objective sensation measures such as 2-point discrimination, monofilament threshold, or vibration testing. Progressive deterioration requires urgent intervention.[4]

Tourniquets are avoided before hospitalization and emergency management to maintain perfusion to surrounding muscle and other soft tissues. Open wounds are irrigated and dressed, with pressure dressings applied to actively bleeding wounds. Extremities are realigned and splinted with adequate analgesia and sedation. Tetanus and antibiotic prophylaxis is given at the time of initial evaluation. First-generation cephalosporin coverage is sufficient for Gustilo-Anderson grade

1 and 2 injuries, and infectious complication rates are more similar to those of closed injuries.[5] For grade 3 injuries, gram-negative coverage with gentamicin is recommended.[5,6] Soil contamination may be an indication for penicillin prophylaxis against clostridia species, and other antibiotics may be recommended for specific scenarios such as aquatic injuries.[6,7]

Plain film radiographs of the wrist and forearm are obtained, including posteroanterior, lateral, and oblique views. A detailed description of the radiological evaluation of distal radius fractures is beyond the scope of this article, but an excellent discussion of this is available elsewhere.[8] Radiographs of the elbow and shoulder are obtained when there is suspicion of proximal injury. Traction and/or stress radiographs may be helpful in identifying fracture fragments and patterns of instability. CT clarifies fracture pattern and position in suspected die punch fractures, volar rim fractures, and carpal fractures or dislocations, but can be difficult to interpret prior to realignment of the injury.

The patient may then be brought to the operating room for surgical debridement, skeletal stabilization, and possible definitive fixation of the fracture and/or soft tissue reconstruction as needed. Physical examination and imaging that were limited by pain and other factors in the emergency department can be better assessed under anesthesia.

SOFT TISSUE MANAGEMENT—LISTER'S TUMOR DEBRIDEMENT

The outcome of open distal radius fractures with significant soft tissue injury is dominated by factors related to the wounds.[5,6] The ability to prevent contamination from becoming sepsis correlates best with functional outcome, and is influenced by the extent and adequacy of debridement and the restoration of the soft tissue envelope.[5,6,9] Historically, tissues were debrided every 48 to 72 hours to allow tissues to declare themselves, until all nonviable tissues were removed.[10,11] This technique is well established, but associated with bacterial wound colonization and delays in definitive reconstruction.[10–12] The authors avoid this wait-and-see approach and perform early aggressive debridement (Box 2).

Lister asserted that upon completion of a single aggressive debridement, the wound should resemble a tumor resection.[12] This is done under tourniquet control, so the viability or ischemia of tissues is not obscured by blood in the field.[12] If the investing tissue of nerves, arteries, and tendons is visibly contaminated, debridement is limited to removal of adventitia, epineurium, and epitenon; excision of intact nerves, arteries, or

---

Box 2
Debridement of open wounds associated with complex distal radius fractures

Restore length with sterile traction set-up or external fixator so that the tissues can be adequately visualized and debrided.

The use of a tourniquet at the time of initial debridement may allow for better visualization of the tissues, limiting the blood in the field.

Early aggressive debridement involves excision of all open contaminated or devascularized tissue except nerves, arteries, and tendons. Lister referred to this as a tumor debridement. This reduces wound colonization and facilitates early soft tissue reconstruction.

Alternatively, wounds can undergo serial debridement every 48 to 72 hours until all tissues have declared themselves. This is a well-established technique, and it remains advantageous for broad crush-type injuries where the extent of soft tissue injury is unclear.

Skeletal stabilization is a critical component of debridement and prevention of infection.

Negative-pressure wound therapy can be used prior to definitive reconstruction, and may minimize wound colonization.

Generally the aim should be to achieve soft tissue reconstruction within 1 week of injury, where possible.

---

tendons is avoided.[12] Tissues are left in place to declare themselves only in the setting of a broad crush injury, where the extent of muscle damage cannot be defined, and this requires repeat debridement every 48 hours.[12]

Free tissue transfer can significantly improve potential for limb salvage over amputation when needed.[13] In cases where immediate soft tissue coverage is not feasible due to available resources or fatigue of the operative team, wet-to-moist gauze can be changed regularly, or polymethylmethacrylate (PMMA) antibiotic bead pouches or negative pressure wound therapy can be applied.[14,15] Generally, the authors aim for complete coverage within 1 week of injury.

The authors often use negative-pressure wound therapy (NPWT) when soft tissue reconstruction is not immediately feasible. Animal data suggest that the negative pressure leads to decreased edema, improved blood flow, increased granulation tissue, and improved bacterial clearance.[16] A recent comparative study of NPWT and wet-to-moist gauze for complex open fracture wounds also showed decreased rates of infection (5.4% vs 28%).[15] On the other hand, NPWT has not been

shown to shorten the time to closure or influence the choice of closure.[15] Size, grade of soft tissue injury, and degree of contamination remain the primary determinants of time to achievement of a clean stable wound for closure, not the dressing.[15]

Prolonged duration of antibiotic coverage has not been shown to improve outcome in regard to infectious complications.[17] A short course of antibiotics (12 hours) has been shown to be equally effective to a prolonged course of antibiotics (14 days).[17] The authors typically limit antibiotic prophylaxis to 24 hours after soft tissue coverage is achieved.

INDIRECT REDUCTION AND SKELETAL STABILIZATION

Realignment of the fracture and skeletal stabilization is a critical component of soft tissue management.[2,3] This can be achieved with external, percutaneous, or internal plate fixation as needed. The authors use a reduction method based on multiplanar ligamentotaxis, as described by Agee, which involves sequential manual traction, palmar translation, and pronation of the hand relative to the forearm.[18] Wrist flexion and forearm pronation are avoided. Five to 10 pounds of axial traction through finger traps aid intraoperative reduction maintenance. Excessive traction is associated with persistent pain, stiffness, and nerve dysfunction.[19]

Fluoroscopic imaging during reduction allows assessment of mechanical alignment, articular congruity, and patterns of instability. Detailed assessment can be obtained when images are taken in multiple planes. In a normal wrist, the lunate facet is inclined approximately 10°, so elevating the forearm 10° from the plane of the receiver plate for the lateral view aids in visualizing the articular surface.[8] The authors center much of their operative decision making on the findings at the time of this closed reduction, and this has largely obviated the need for a preoperative CT scan.

Although the current trend is to prefer open reduction and internal fixation to percutaneous and external fixation for distal radius fractures, bridging external fixation remains well suited for complex injuries.[3,20] External fixators can retain length, allow soft tissue management, and temporarily stabilize fractures when immediate definitive care is not feasible. Complications include superficial radial nerve injury, pin tract infection, and loss of reduction, but these can be prevented with open incisions and blunt dissection, loose pin site closure, and additional percutaneous pin fixation to prevent loss of articular reduction.[19–21]

The authors' preferred variation on the concept of external fixation is the spanning internal fixator or distal radius bridge plate. The concept was first described by Burke and Singer, and has since been modified by Ruch and Hanel.[22–25] A locking plate is passed under the extensor retinaculum using limited incisions proximally and distally, and is fixed to the radial and metacarpal diaphyses.[22–25] The authors use a 2.4/2.7 mm stainless steel plate specifically designed for use as a distal radius bridge plate (DRB plate, Synthes, Paoli, Pennsylvania), passed through the second dorsal compartment.[25]

Compared with external fixation, the dorsal bridge plate technique avoids pin tract infection, reduces nursing care, and provides strong fixation immediately adjacent to bone.[19,22–25] It can be combined with a limited open articular fixation approach as needed. If reduction is satisfactory and well maintained, the plate is removed following adequate fracture healing. This usually takes about 4 months (especially for open injuries), and is followed by wrist rehabilitation.[23] The plate can also be used like a temporary external fixator, with removal at the time of definitive osteosynthesis or soft tissue reconstruction. Wrist range-of-motion and upper limb functional scores are not significantly related to duration of plate fixation at 1 year postoperatively for patients treated with the dorsal bridge plate.[23]

FUNCTIONAL ANATOMY AND OPERATIVE TACTIC—THE COLUMN MODEL

The authors' preferred framework for osseoligamentous management of complex distal radius fractures is the columnar concept of Rikli and Regazzoni, which describes the wrist in terms of 3 columns: the lateral (or radial) column, the intermediate column, and the medial (or ulnar) column.[2,3] Understanding wrist anatomy and typical patterns of fracture aids in prioritizing goals and determining the sequence of surgical intervention. Even in extremely comminuted fractures where immediate or delayed wrist fusion is considered, preservation of soft tissues and normal anatomic relationships maximizes forearm rotation and hand function.

The Lateral Column

The lateral (or radial) column is composed of radial styloid and scaphoid facet. Counter to historical cadaveric studies, it is not a principal weight-bearing surface in vivo.[26] It serves as a ligamentous attachment for the carpus and a buttress against carpal translation radially, particularly during radioulnar deviation.[26] The radioscaphocapitate and radial collateral ligaments attach the lateral column to the carpus volarly and radially.

At the time of injury, the distal radius often splits between the scaphoid and lunate facets, and scaphoid fossa articular fractures tend to occur at the central and ulnar aspects dorsally (**Fig. 1**).[27] Reduction of the styloid is focused more on translation in the coronal and sagittal planes than on tilt or articular congruity. Percutaneous axial Kirschner wire fixation is often a reasonable provisional fixation. It may be combined with indirect means to maintain reduction such as intraoperative finger-trap traction, an external fixator, or a dorsal bridge plate. Gap between the scaphoid and lunate

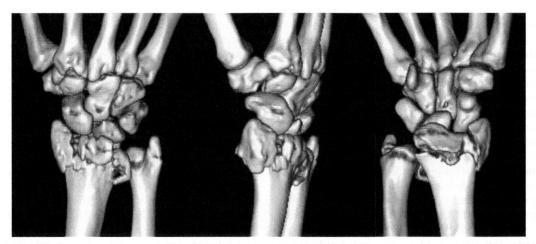

Fig. 1. A 3-dimensional representation of a high-energy distal radius fracture. The radius is split between the scaphoid and lunate facets. The volar rim fragment is dorsiflexed. There is articular comminution centrally on the dorsal rim. The attachments of the dorsal and volar radioulnar ligaments are split at the sigmoid notch, and the anteroposterior distance is widened.

ossae should be avoided to decrease stress on the scapholunate ligaments. The brachioradialis inserts on the radial aspect and may be released during open exposure to decrease deforming forces.

Definitive fixation for the radial column varies. In many cases, provisional percutaneous Kirschner wires may be left in place for 3 to 4 weeks, or longer if cut below the skin. Screw fixation has the advantage of providing additional stability and less soft tissue prominence. A volar plate with multiple fixed angle screws, including 1 or 2 screws into the styloid, is often satisfactory once adequate reduction has been achieved. Low-profile plates and pin-and-plate constructs have also been used.[3,8] The benefit of open exposure is balanced against the potential for local scar and unsuccessful reduction and fixation. In cases where there is significant comminution, the styloid should be reformed into the general shape of its native alignment and fixed as best as possible.

The Intermediate Column

The intermediate column is the primary load-bearing column of the wrist and a focus for evaluation of mechanical alignment, articular congruity, and translational stability.[2,3,26] It includes both the lunate facet and the sigmoid notch, and has strong attachments to the lunate volarly and the triquetrum dorsally, which are important in carpal translational stability and motion. Dorsal and volar radiolunar ligaments attach the ulna to the sigmoid notch and are important for normal forearm rotation. Fractures commonly occur between ligamentous attachments at the center of the sigmoid notch and between the short and long radiolunate ligaments of the lunate fossa (see Fig. 1).[27]

Restoration of length and palmar tilt of the intermediate column is a first priority for mechanical alignment, and is the foundation for further reduction and fixation. This is done with reduction and traction, and possibly percutaneous reduction techniques with pins or small instruments. Increased ulnar variance can cause significant symptomatic ulnocarpal impaction, and the DRUJ becomes incongruous with a characteristic loss of forearm rotation.[28,29] Loss or over-reduction of volar tilt also can alter DRUJ ligament mechanics and explain loss of forearm rotation for some patients.[28,29]

Intermediate column articular congruity is addressed simultaneously with mechanical alignment, but fine adjustments can also be made after gross mechanical alignment is achieved. Fracture step and gap are commonly cited factors

in predicting later arthrosis,[30] but arc of congruity is also important to assess.[8] The volar rim fragment may be dorsiflexed or anteroposterior distance widened, and the smooth arc of rotation may no longer be present.[8] This results in increased contact pressures, articular shear, and arthrosis. On a true lateral view, the radiographic axis of the volar rim fragment should be approximately 70° to the longitudinal axis of the radius.[8]

Translational instability at time of initial reduction is important in determining surgical approach and implant placement. The carpus and volar rim segment typically move together due to strong ligament attachments (Figs. 2 and 3). In cases where there is volar translation or failure to reduce a volar rim fragment with traction and indirect techniques, a volar buttress is essential to avoid later displacement. Care should be taken to avoid plate prominence over the volar lip, as this may lead to attritional tendon rupture. When complete, there should be colinearity of the volar cortex of the radial diaphysis, the center of the lunate, and the center of the capitate.[8]

Familiarity with various open exposures of the wrist is a prerequisite for management of complex injuries. The flexor carpi radialis (FCR) approach is a workhorse approach, extensile proximally, for both the intermediate and lateral columns. Distal extension to the carpal tunnel risks injury to the palmar cutaneous branch, so a separate carpal tunnel incision should be used when needed. An alternative is the volar ulnar approach, which involves dissection between the ulnar neurovascular bundle and the contents of the carpal tunnel, then incision through pronator quadratus. This can be extended distally to release the carpal tunnel and provides excellent exposure of the volar ulnar corner of the radius. The pronator quadratus is typically not repairable at closure. Open dorsal approaches to the intermediate column may utilize the third compartment, fifth compartment, or 3,4 or 4,5 intervals. Open dorsal approaches share in common the need to avoid injuring important radiocarpal or DRUJ ligament structures, plate prominence under tendons, or stripping the dorsoulnar fragment of soft tissue attachments.

Ultimately, reduction and fixation depend on several factors. The balance is weighed between rigid fracture stability and secondary soft tissue insult and scarring. If debridement is thorough, and early or immediate soft tissue coverage provided, placing fixation through existing wounds is advantageous. Otherwise, indirect reduction and spanning fixation (ie, with a dorsal spanning wrist plate) or a single open exposure and volar or dorsal locking plate of adequate length may be desirable.[21] Additional percutaneous fixation

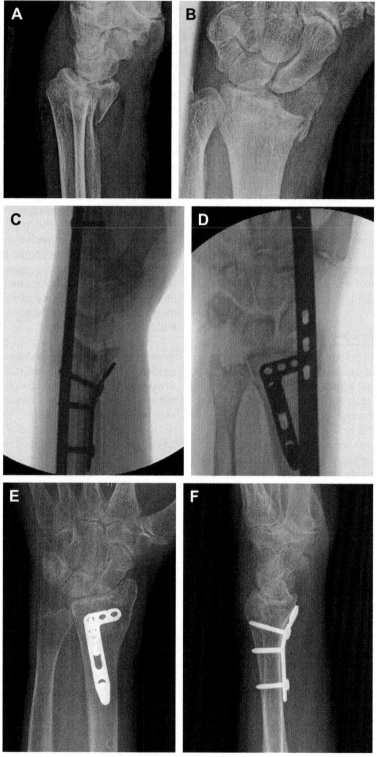

Fig. 2. A 70-year-old woman sustained a comminuted distal radius fracture, with volar and dorsal intermediate column fragments and comminution of the radial column. (*A, B*) There was a volar shear component with translation of the carpus. Length was maintained with intraoperative traction, and a volar ulnar approach was used to reduce the articular fragments through the fracture. (*C, D*) A 2.7 mm buttress plate was used to maintain position of the volar rim, and a 2.7 mm dorsal spanning plate was used to maintain length and palmar tilt until removal 4 months after injury. (*E, F*) Radiographs show the healed position of the fracture.

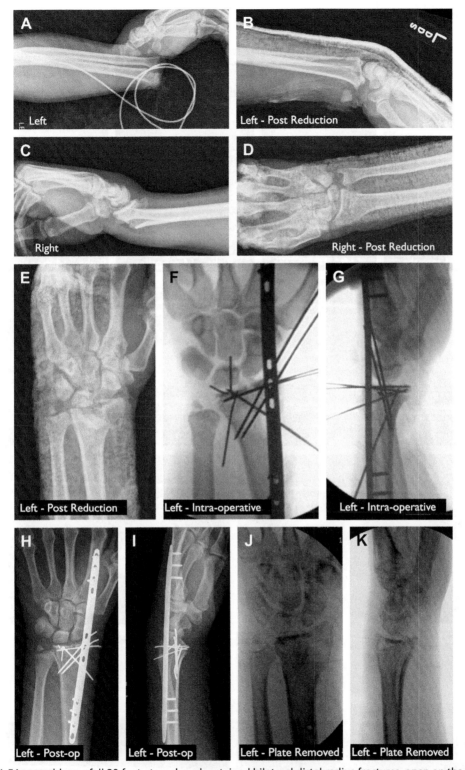

Fig. 3. A 54-year-old man fell 20 feet at work and sustained bilateral distal radius fractures, open on the left side (Gustilo 2). (*A*) The fractures were grossly reduced and splinted prior to transfer. (*A–E*) Intraoperatively, the open wound was debrided, including a free bone fragment that was removed from the volar tissues (seen in *B*). This was determined to be a portion of the lunate facet. A volar FCR approach was combined with a dorsal approach to the wrist to obtain reduction of the multiple articular pieces. The free fragment of lunate facet was fixed in a reduced position with the other fragments using Kirschner wires. (*F, G*) Postoperative views showed maintained alignment with application of the dorsal spanning plate to neutralize forces across the wrist. (*H, I*) The plate was later removed (*J, K*), and alignment was maintained at 14 months. (*L, M*) The right wrist was fixed with a volar locking plate. (*N, O*) At 14 months he has mild pain with strenuous activity with the left wrist, but is otherwise satisfied and has good range of motion (*P–U*).

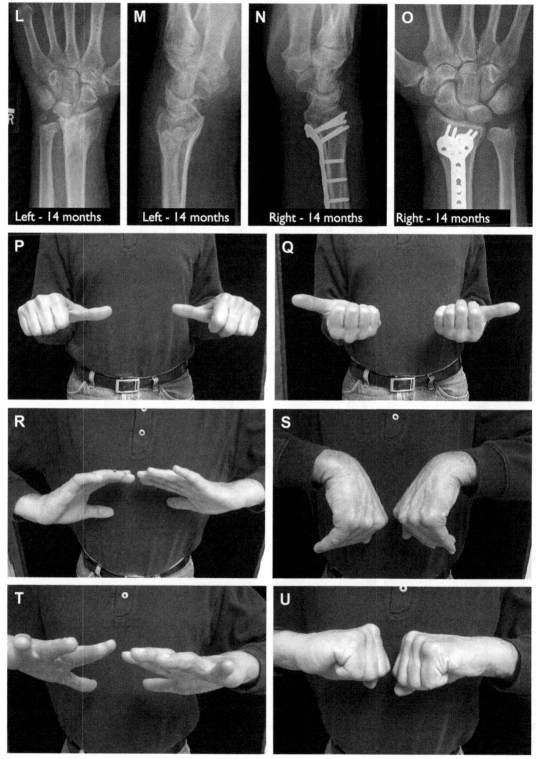

L   Left - 14 months
M   Left - 14 months
N   Right - 14 months
O   Right - 14 months

Fig. 3. (*continued*)

can provide adequate further fixation if needed. Low-profile volar or dorsal plating is an option for displaced fragments that cannot be otherwise fixed with pins or screws, but poor bone quality and comminution may also preclude adequate fixation even despite open exposure.

The Medial Column

The medial column is the rotational center of the wrist.[2,3] It includes the distal ulna and triangular fibrocartilage complex (TFCC), which stabilize wrist and forearm rotation and other wrist motion.[2,3] Ulnar-sided discomfort and loss of forearm supination are the most common sources of persistent symptoms after distal radius fracture.[31]

The triangular fibrocartilage complex (TFCC) inserts on the fovea centralis and ulnar styloid of the ulna. Cadaveric studies have shown that disruption of the TFCC and/or ulnar styloid base fracture occurs with shortening the radius as little as 5 mm.[28] However, provided that the distal radius is anatomically reduced, fixation of ulnar styloid fractures is generally not required and does not improve outcome, even in cases involving at least three-fourths of the height of the styloid.[32] A comparison of direct repair of the ulnar styloid versus immobilization of the forearm in 60° of supination in patients treated with external fixators found that immobilization in supination resulted in better supination and fewer complications.[32] Management of medial column injury, therefore, is generally done after the lateral and intermediate columns have been addressed.

If the DRUJ is stable after radius fixation but there was evidence of ulnar styloid fracture or other DRUJ injury, the authors immobilize the limb in a long-arm splint with the forearm in supination for the first 10 to 14 days postoperatively. If the DRUJ is unstable and there are no contraindications to prolonging the operation, repair or reconstruction of the DRUJ and TFCC is undertaken. If the patient's condition does not allow the operation to be prolonged, the ulnar head can be reduced manually into the sigmoid notch and the ulna transfixed to the radius with a minimum of 2 1.6 mm Kirschner wires passed proximal to the DRUJ.

The Pedestal

Although strictly not a component of the Rikli and Regazzoni framework, it is also important to consider metadiaphyseal stability and bone loss, the pedestal of the intermediate and lateral columns. Complex fractures of the distal radius are commonly associated with bone loss, either due to actual loss of bone or as a consequence of significant impaction resulting in a localized void of structural support. Insertion of autogenous bone graft has been shown to produce improvements in healing time, radiographic results, and functional outcome scores.[33]

Autogenous graft has the benefits of osteogenesis, osteoinduction, osteoconduction, structural support, and incorporation/remodeling into normal bone. It remains the gold standard for treatment of local bone defects, but is associated with donor site morbidity and complications.[33–36] Allograft bone has been used as an alternative, but lacks the same osteogenic and osteoinductive properties, and carries a remote risk of disease transmission.[33–36]

In recent years, numerous substitutes have been developed as alternatives to bone graft.[33,36] Recent reviews written by Nauth and colleagues[36] and Ladd and colleagues[33] discuss the various biologic, mechanical, handling, and resorption properties of available products. Unfortunately, there are a limited number of clinical studies, and most lack direct comparison between products.

Despite new products, the goals for treatment remain the same, and are dependent on the location and size of the defect. Bone grafts and substitutes are an adjunct and do not replace operative stabilization. Small metaphyseal voids with adequate subchondral support of the articular surface do not require additional treatment, and will consolidate with time.[33,36] Larger metaphyseal defects with limited support of the articular surface, such as a die punch fragment, may benefit from bone graft or substitutes with high initial compressive strength properties and osteoconduction (eg, cancellous allograft, calcium phosphate, coralline hydroxyapatite).[33,36] Osteoinduction and osteogenesis are not required in metaphyseal fractures, because these well-vascularized defects will heal spontaneously.[36] The authors' preference remains to use dried morcellized cancellous allograft for such defects.

Diaphyseal bone loss is in an area of higher shear stresses and torsional loads and tends to have poorer rates of healing.[33,36] A greater degree of structural support is needed, as well as osteogenic and/or osteoinductive potential.[33,36] Open exposure and grafting are balanced against indirect reduction and spanning fixation. When voids remain, autogenous iliac crest bone graft remains the gold standard, and cancellous allograft can be mixed with it to act as an extender for its osteoconductive and structural properties.[33,36] Calcium phosphate cement lacks the tensile strength and osteoinductivity required for this location.[36] In cases of large segmental bone defects, options include large amounts of bone graft, acute shortening of the radius and ulna, bone transport, vascularized bone transfer, or an induced membranes technique.[36]

CARPAL INSTABILITY

Carpal instability is frequently associated with distal radius fractures. Scapholunate interosseous ligament tears have been observed in 18% to 64% of distal radius fractures in some series, and lunotriquetral tears in 12% to 16% of distal radius fractures when evaluated arthroscopically.[37–40] Scaphoid and other carpal fractures may also be present. Vigilance is required to identify clinical and radiographic abnormalities suggestive of a tear, fracture, or in some cases even perilunate dislocation. An advantage to traction imaging is the better ability to identify features of carpal instability such as disruption of Gilula lines or scapholunate widening. A scaphoid ring or signet ring sign may also be seen with the scaphoid flexed and the tuberosity superimposed on the waist. Fortunately, some forms of instability and malalignment are treated by addressing the distal radius fracture.

Persistent instability evidenced on traction fluoroscopy is best treated by open reduction and intercarpal pinning, either alone or in combination with ligament repair, debridement, capsulodesis, or ligament reconstruction.[41,42] Closed reduction and percutaneous fixation are only acceptable if anatomic reduction is achieved and maintained. A missed diagnosis of perilunate dislocation or closed treatment without additional stabilization leads to uniformly poor results.[41] Delays in reduction lead to increased rates of post-traumatic arthrosis and median neuropathy.[41,43]

OUTCOME

Outcome after complex distal radius fracture is a function of multiple factors. Limb survival is largely dependent on management of acute neurovascular injury, compartment syndrome, and avoidance of infection.[9] Wrist and forearm range of motion and objective impairment are influenced more by adequacy of restoration of osseoligamentous relationships and minimization of scar.

More recently, it has also been recognized that outcome of injuries such as these is also significantly influenced by psychosocial influences. Post-traumatic stress disorder (PTSD) and clinically relevant depression have been reported to approach prevalence of 51% and 45%, respectively in orthopedic fracture clinics, and this can outweigh objective impairments for patients.[44,45] Ring and colleagues[46] found depression to be the strongest predictor of poor upper extremity function for multiple diagnoses, including distal radius

fractures. Worker's compensation status is also a strong negative predictor of functional status, as is pain catastrophizing.[46,47] Screening can often be completed in a short amount of time,[48] and psychological symptoms may be treated with psychotherapy and/or pharmacologic treatment.[49]

SUMMARY

The comprehensive management of complex distal radius fractures requires a thorough understanding of wrist functional anatomy and familiarity with a wide selection of approaches and fixation options. Treatment must be adapted to the soft tissue injury, fracture pattern, and patient considerations. Outcome is determined by multiple factors and depends greatly on the soft tissue management and restoration of osseoligamentous relationships. The psychosocial health of the patient is emerging as an important factor in functional outcome.

REFERENCES

1. Court-Brown CM, Caesar B. Epidemiology of adult fractures: a review. Injury 2006;37(8):691–7.
2. Rikli DA, Regazzoni P. Fractures of the distal end of the radius treated by internal fixation and early function. A preliminary report of 20 cases. J Bone Joint Surg Br 1996;78(4):588–92.
3. Rikli DA, Rosenkranz J, Regazzoni P. Complex fractures of the distal radius. Eur J Trauma 2003;29(4): 199–207.
4. Mack GR, McPherson SA, Lutz RB. Acute median neuropathy after wrist trauma. The role of emergent carpal tunnel release. Clin Orthop Relat Res 1994; 300:141–6.
5. Gustilo RB, Anderson JT. Prevention of infection in the treatment of one thousand and twenty-five open fractures of long bones: retrospective and prospective analyses. J Bone Joint Surg Am 1976;58(4):453–8.
6. Sanders R, Swiontkowski M, Nunley J, et al. The management of fractures with soft-tissue disruptions. J Bone Joint Surg Am 1993;75(5):778–89.
7. Noonburg GE. Management of extremity trauma and related infections occurring in the aquatic environment. J Am Acad Orthop Surg 2005;13(4):243–53.
8. Medoff RJ. Essential radiographic evaluation for distal radius fractures. Hand Clin 2005;21(3):279–88.
9. Axelrod TS, Buchler U. Severe complex injuries to the upper extremity: revascularization and replantation. J Hand Surg Am 1991;16(4):574–84.
10. Haury B, Rodeheaver G, Vensko J, et al. Debridement: an essential component of traumatic wound care. Am J Surg 1978;135(2):238–42.
11. Burkhalter WE, Butler B, Metz W, et al. Experiences with delayed primary closure of war wounds of the

hand in Viet Nam. J Bone Joint Surg Am 1968;50(5): 945–54.

2. Lister GD. Emergency free flaps. In: Green DP, editor. Operative hand surgery. Edinburgh (Scotland): Churchill-Livingstone; 1988. p. 1127–49.

3. Lister G, Scheker L. Emergency free flaps to the upper extremity. J Hand Surg Am 1988;13(1):22–8.

4. Keating JF, Blachut PA, O'Brien PJ, et al. Reamed nailing of open tibial fractures: does the antibiotic bead pouch reduce the deep infection rate? J Orthop Trauma 1996;10(5):298–303.

5. Stannard JP, Volgas DA, Stewart R, et al. Negative pressure wound therapy after severe open fractures: a prospective randomized study. J Orthop Trauma 2009;23(8):552–7.

6. Orgill DP, Bayer LR. Update on negative-pressure wound therapy. Plast Reconstr Surg 2011;127(Suppl 1): 105S–15S.

7. Dellinger EP. Antibiotic prophylaxis in trauma: penetrating abdominal injuries and open fractures. Rev Infect Dis 1991;13(Suppl 10):S847–57.

8. Agee JM. Distal radius fractures. Multiplanar ligamentotaxis. Hand Clin 1993;9(4):577–85.

9. Diaz-Garcia RJ, Oda T, Shauver MJ, et al. A systematic review of outcomes and complications of treating unstable distal radius fractures in the elderly. J Hand Surg Am 2011;36(5):824–35.e2.

20. Koval KJ, Harrast JJ, Anglen JO, et al. Fractures of the distal part of the radius. The evolution of practice over time. Where's the evidence? J Bone Joint Surg Am 2008;90(9):1855–61.

21. Wolfe SW, Swigart CR, Grauer J, et al. Augmented external fixation of distal radius fractures: a biomechanical analysis. J Hand Surg Am 1998;23(1): 127–34.

22. Burke EF, Singer RM. Treatment of comminuted distal radius with the use of an internal distraction plate. Tech Hand Up Extrem Surg 1998;2(4):248–52.

23. Ruch DS, Ginn TA, Yang CC, et al. Use of a distraction plate for distal radial fractures with metaphyseal and diaphyseal comminution. J Bone Joint Surg Am 2005;87(5):945–54.

24. Ginn TA, Ruch DS, Yang CC, et al. Use of a distraction plate for distal radial fractures with metaphyseal and diaphyseal comminution. Surgical technique. J Bone Joint Surg Am 2006;88(Suppl 1 Pt 1):29–36.

25. Wolf J, Weil W, Hanel D, et al. A biomechanic comparison of an internal radiocarpal-spanning 2.4-mm locking plate and external fixation in a model of distal radius fractures. J Hand Surg Am 2006;31(10):1578–86.

26. Rikli DA, Honigmann P, Babst R, et al. Intra-articular pressure measurement in the radioulnocarpal joint using a novel sensor: in vitro and in vivo results. J Hand Surg Am 2007;32(1):67–75.

27. Mandziak DG, Watts AC, Bain GI. Ligament contribution to patterns of articular fractures of the distal radius. J Hand Surg Am 2011;36(10):1621–5.

28. Adams BD. Effects of radial deformity on distal radioulnar joint mechanics. J Hand Surg Am 1993; 18(3):492–8.

29. Crisco JJ, Moore DC, Marai GE, et al. Effects of distal radius malunion on distal radioulnar joint mechanics—an in vivo study. J Orthop Res 2007;25(4):547–55.

30. Knirk JL, Jupiter JB. Intra-articular fractures of the distal end of the radius in young adults. J Bone Joint Surg Am 1986;68(5):647–59.

31. Tsukazaki T, Iwasaki K. Ulnar wrist pain after Colles' fracture. 109 fractures followed for 4 years. Acta Orthop Scand 1993;64(4):462–4.

32. Ruch DS, Lumsden BC, Papadonikolakis A. Distal radius fractures: a comparison of tension band wiring versus ulnar outrigger external fixation for the management of distal radioulnar instability. J Hand Surg Am 2005;30(5):969–77.

33. Ladd AL, Pliam NB. The role of bone graft and alternatives in unstable distal radius fracture treatment. Orthop Clin North Am 2001;32(2):337–51.

34. Seiler JG, Johnson J. Iliac crest autogenous bone grafting: donor site complications. J South Orthop Assoc 2000;9(2):91–7.

35. Myeroff C, Archdeacon M. Autogenous bone graft: donor sites and techniques. J Bone Joint Surg Am 2011;93(23):2227–36.

36. Nauth A, McKee MD, Einhorn TA, et al. Managing bone defects. J Orthop Trauma 2011;25(8):462–6.

37. Forward DP, Lindau TR, Melsom DS. Intercarpal ligament injuries associated with fractures of the distal part of the radius. J Bone Joint Surg Am 2007; 89(11):2334–40.

38. Richards RS, Bennett JD, Roth JH, et al. Arthroscopic diagnosis of intra-articular soft tissue injuries associated with distal radial fractures. J Hand Surg Am 1997;22(5):772–6.

39. Lindau T, Arner M, Hagberg L. Intraarticular lesions in distal fractures of the radius in young adults. A descriptive arthroscopic study in 50 patients. J Hand Surg Br 1997;22(5):638–43.

40. Geissler WB, Freeland AE, Savoie FH, et al. Intracarpal soft-tissue lesions associated with an intraarticular fracture of the distal end of the radius. J Bone Joint Surg Am 1996;78(3):357–65.

41. Herzberg G, Comtet JJ, Linscheid RL, et al. Perilunate dislocations and fracture-dislocations: a multicenter study. J Hand Surg Am 1993;18:768–79.

42. Zarkadas PC, Gropper PT, White NJ, et al. A survey of the surgical management of acute and chronic scapholunate instability. J Hand Surg Am 2004; 29(5):848–57.

43. Inoue G, Shionoya K. Late treatment of unreduced perilunate dislocations. J Hand Surg Br 1999;24(2): 221–5.

44. Starr AJ, Smith WR, Frawley WH, et al. Symptoms of posttraumatic stress disorder after orthopaedic trauma. J Bone Joint Surg Am 2004;86(6):1115–21.

45. Crichlow RJ, Andres PL, Morrison SM, et al. Depression in orthopaedic trauma patients. Prevalence and severity. J Bone Joint Surg Am 2006;88(9):1927–33.

46. Ring D, Kadzielski J, Fabian L, et al. Self-reported upper extremity health status correlates with depression. J Bone Joint Surg Am 2006;88(9):1983–8.

47. Grewal R, Macdermid JC, Pope J, et al. Baseline predictors of pain and disability one year following extra-articular distal radius fractures. Hand (N Y) 2007;2(3):104–11.

48. Grunert BK, Hargarten SW, Matloub HS, et al. Predictive value of psychological screening in acute hand injuries. J Bone Joint Surg Am 1992;17(2):196–9.

49. Vranceanu AM, Barsky A, Ring D. Psychosocial aspects of disabling musculoskeletal pain. J Bone Joint Surg Am 2009;91(8):2014–8.

Fracture-Dislocations of the Carpus: Perilunate Injury

Prasad J. Sawardeker, MD, MS[a], Katie E. Kindt, BS[a],
Mark E. Baratz, MD[b],*

KEYWORDS

• Perilunate • Carpal instability • Fracture-dislocation

KEY POINTS

• Perilunate injuries are rare; unfortunately, the consequences of improper recognition and inappropriate management can be debilitating.
• Injuries occur as a result of a high-energy load leading to carpal disruption and progressive ligamentous and bone injury.
• Loss of motion, diminished grip strength and post-traumatic arthrosis are common consequences despite appropriate treatment.
• Successful outcomes depend on time to treatment, open or closed nature of the injury, extent of chondral damage, residual instability, and fracture union.

INTRODUCTION

Perilunate injuries are rare; unfortunately, the consequences of improper recognition and inappropriate management can be debilitating. Injuries occur as a result of a high-energy load leading to carpal disruption and progressive ligamentous and bone injury. The most commonly described events include falls, sports-related injuries, and motorcycle and motor vehicle accidents. Mayfield and colleagues[1] observed that cadaveric wrists loaded in hyperextension, ulnar deviation, and carpal supination reproduced the injury. Progressive failure of ligament and bone contributes to predictable patterns with multiple variants. Injuries are divided into *perilunate dislocations* and *perilunate fracture dislocations*. Deformity can sometimes be subtle, and spontaneous reduction has been reported.[2,3] Prompt recognition is a challenge, and up to 25% of these injuries are missed on initial presentation.[4] Early and accurate diagnosis is critical to prevent progressive pain and dysfunction.[4] Treatment involves an attempt at closed reduction followed by surgical intervention to restore carpal alignment and stability. Delay is associated with poor outcomes, including post-traumatic arthritis, decreased motion and grip strength, median nerve impairment, disability, loss of wages, and even attritional rupture of flexor tendons.[5] This article reviews carpal anatomy and kinematics, classification systems, treatment options, and expected outcomes.

WRIST BIOMECHANICS

The wrist is a diarthrodial joint comprised of 8 carpal bones arranged in 2 rows. The geometry of the carpal bones and their attachments allows motion in 2 primary planes: flexion-extension and radio-ulnar deviation. The flexion-extension arc is derived from roughly equal motion through the radiocarpal articulation and the midcarpal articulation. Radio-ulnar deviation is similarly distributed with the radiocarpal joint contributing 40% and the midcarpal joint contributing 60%.[6]

Disclosures: Nothing to disclose.
[a] Orthopedic Surgery Department, Allegheny General Hospital, 1307 Federal Street, 2nd Floor, Pittsburgh, PA 15212, USA; [b] Hand and Upper Extremity Service, Department of Orthopedic Surgery, Allegheny General Hospital, Drexel University, 1307 Federal Street, 2nd Floor, Pittsburgh, PA 15212, USA
* Corresponding author.
E-mail address: mbaratz@wpahs.org

Orthop Clin N Am 44 (2013) 93–106
http://dx.doi.org/10.1016/j.ocl.2012.08.009

There are several theories to explain carpal kinematics and function. Bryce[7] described carpal bone motion based on radiographs of his own wrist. Since then, several tools have been used to evaluate wrist motion, including uniplanar radiographs,[8] measurement of inserted wires into individual carpal bones,[9] fluoroscopy,[10] cineradiography,[11] stereoscopic measurement,[12] light emitting diodes,[13] and 3-dimensional computed tomographic (CT) imaging.[14]

In the early twentieth century, Navarro[15] proposed that the carpus was arranged in 3 rigid, vertical columns. The central column (lunate and capitate) provided a base for axial loading. The medial column (triquetrum, pisiform, and hamate) created a pivot point around which the carpus could rotate. The lateral column (scaphoid, trapezium, and trapezoid) acted as a mobile linkage column. Taleisnik[16] modified the 3-column concept in 1976 by including the trapezium and trapezoid in the central column while eliminating the pisiform from the medial column. In 1988, Weber[17] introduced the longitudinal column theory of a force-bearing column and a control column. The force-bearing column bore weight and consisted of the radius, lunate, proximal two-thirds of the scaphoid, capitate, and trapezoid. The control column provided control during motion and was comprised of the ulna, ulnocarpal complex, triquetrum and hamate, and the fourth and fifth metacarpal bases. The column theories provided a model to account for axial load transmission from the hand to forearm; however, they failed to explain the coupled motion between the proximal and distal rows. Additionally, it did not account for the small but significant independent motion present between carpal bones.[13]

The row theory was introduced in the 1980s and suggested that the proximal and distal rows behaved as separate functional units.[6,13,18] The distal row was fixed to the metacarpal bases with very little intercarpal motion, creating a distal hand segment. The forearm comprised the proximal stable segment. The proximal carpal row was the intercalated segment, with freedom of motion caused by the bony configuration and ligamentous attachments. The scaphoid was thought to serve as a linkage and strut mechanism, which maintained the integrity of the intercalated segment under axial loading forces. To their credit, Linscheid and colleagues,[19] years earlier, recognized that no muscles or tendons insert on the proximal carpal row and, as a result, proposed that the scaphoid, lunate, and triquetrum acted as an intercalated segment between the rigid distal carpal row and the radius and ulna.[19] The interosseous ligaments between the bones and the articular geometry allowed them to move in unison during wrist motion.

Linscheid and Weber observed carpal motion in the radial-ulnar plane and formulated different theories on the mechanics involved. Linscheid[20] noted that as the wrist radially deviates, the scaphoid and proximal row flex. He thought that scaphoid flexion occurred in response to the pressure exerted by the trapezium and trapezoid. Weber[17] postulated that it was the helicoid geometry of the triquetrohamate articulation that forced the distal row to translate palmarly during radial deviation. Volar translation of the distal row placed a flexion moment on the proximal row causing it to rotate into flexion.

Different theories on kinematics have offered a greater understanding of the coordinated motion between rows and the tendencies for motion when the system breaks down. Gifford and colleagues[21] took note of the flexion and extension arcs of motion at the wrist and the relative contributions from the radiolunate and lunocapitate articulations. They thought that each row rotated around a single axis of rotation located around its proximal articular surface. They observed the instability of the arrangement and thought that the scaphoid was part of both rows and functioned to link the radius and the distal carpus, offering stability to an otherwise unstable system. Lichtman and colleagues[22–24] initially introduced the oval ring concept; they thought that the circular arrangement of ligaments provided a continuum of stability and allowed for reciprocal motion between the proximal and distal rows. The rows are linked by the scaphotrapezial joint (mobile radial link) and the triquetrohamate joint (rotatory ulnar link).

No one concept adequately describes the complexity of carpal motion, and most agree that carpal kinetics can be explained by a combination of theories. It is evident that in the intact wrist, a balanced synchrony exists between the carpal bones and between the proximal row and distal row.

LIGAMENT ANATOMY AND MECHANICS

Intrinsic ligaments and extrinsic ligaments of the wrist link and stabilize the carpal bones (Fig. 1). Intrinsic ligaments, otherwise known as interosseous ligaments, connect carpal bones to one another. Extrinsic ligaments connect the carpal bones to the radius and ulna and tend to be stronger than their intrinsic counterparts. There are 2 intrinsic interosseous ligaments in the proximal row (scapholunate and lunotriquetral) and 3 within the distal row (deep capitolunate, deep trapeziocapitate, trapeziotrapezoid). Extrinsic ligaments are classified as either volar or dorsal. Dorsal extrinsic ligaments include the dorsal radiocarpal and dorsal intercarpal ligaments. There are

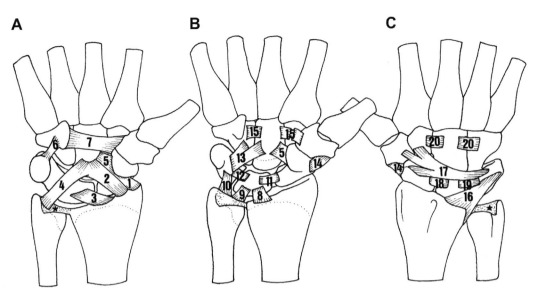

Fig. 1. Schematic representation of the intrinsic and extrinsic ligaments of the wrist. *A.* Palmar superficial ligaments: radioscaphoid (1); radioscaphoid-capitate (2); long radiolunate (3); ulnar capitate (4); scaphoid capitate (5); pisohamate (6); transverse carpal ligament (7). *B.* Palmar deep ligaments: short radiolunate (8); ulnar lunate (9); ulnar triquetrum (10); palmar scapholunate (11); palmar lunate triquetrum (12); triquetral-hamate-capitate (13); dorsolateral STT (14); and palmar transverse interosseous ligaments of the distal row (15). *C.* Dorsal ligaments: radial triquetrum, also referred to as dorsal radiocarpal (16); triquetrum-scaphoid-trapeziotrapezoid, also referred to as dorsal intercarpal (17); dorsal scapholunate (18); dorsal lunate triquetrum (19); and dorsal transverse interosseous ligaments of the distal row (20). Asterisk depicts triangular fibrocartilage. (*From* Garcia-Elias M, Geissler WB. Carpal instability. In: Green DP, Hotchkiss RN, Pederson WC, et al, eds. Green's Operative Hand Surgery, 5th ed. Philadelphia; 2005. p. 535–604; with permission.)

4 volar radiocarpal ligaments (radial collateral, radioscaphocapitate, long radiolunate, and short radiolunate), 4 volar ulnocarpal ligaments (ulnar collateral, ulnotriquetral, ulnolunate, ulnocapitate), and one volar deltoid intercalated ligament. Volar extrinsic ligaments are thicker and stronger than the 2 dorsal extrinsic ligaments. As noted earlier, tendons do not directly insert on the carpals (except the pisiform) but help to stabilize their motion when actively contracting. Wrist motion tends to be initiated by the distal carpal row and metacarpals, which move as a unit. During wrist flexion, the distal row flexes and ulnar deviates. As the distal row flexes, the proximal row flexes. Conversely, with wrist extension, the distal row extends and radially deviates. As the distal row extends, the proximal row extends. Radial deviation of the wrist causes the distal row to incline radially, extend, and supinate, which leads the proximal row to flex and translate in an ulnar direction. During ulnar deviation, the distal row inclines ulnarly, flexes, and pronates causing the proximal row to extend and translate in the radial direction.

CARPAL INSTABILITY

Carpal instability is a broad term that is used to describe the carpal position that results following disruption to bone and/or wrist ligaments. Acute instability usually results from violent trauma, such as a fall or motor vehicle accident. Injury to an interosseous ligament can cause dissociation between carpal bones of a row. The most commonly injured structures are the scapholunate interosseous ligament between the scaphoid and lunate and the lunotriquetral interosseous ligament between the lunate and triquetrum. The thickest region of the scapholunate ligament is dorsal, whereas the lunotriquetral ligament is strongest volarly. Injury to one of these structures leads to altered carpal mechanics, called *carpal instability dissociative.*[25] Disruption that alters motion between the proximal and distal carpal rows has been termed *carpal instability nondissociative.* A ligamentous disruption occurring within a row and between rows has been designated *carpal instability complex.*

PERILUNATE INSTABILITY

Perilunate instability is a type of carpal instability complex. In this case, the carpal anatomy is disrupted in a predictable manner. Progressive ligament and bone dissociation depend on the degree of force imparted on the wrist. The defining feature of the perilunate injury is dissociation of the capitate from the lunate; 95% to 97% are dorsal perilunate dislocations (dorsal displacement of the capitate with respect to the longitudinal axis). Palmar dislocations are quite uncommon and in one series represented only 3% of perilunate injuries.[4] Deformity can be subtle; spontaneous reduction has been reported, making missed injuries common.[2,3]

Progressive perilunar instability was described by Mayfield.[1] Cadaver wrists loaded in wrist extension, ulnar deviation, and intercarpal supination produced a characteristic sequence of carpus disruption around the lunate. Sequential disruption occurs in 4 stages (**Fig. 2**). In stage 1, the scapholunate ligament is disrupted and the radioscapholunate ligament is torn. The force is then transmitted to the lunocapitate articulation where the capitate dislocates. Stage II is accompanied by injury to the radioscaphocapitate ligament, dorsal intercarpal ligament, and radial collateral

ligament. In stage III, energy propagates into the lunotriquetral joint tearing the lunotriquetral ligament. A triquetral dislocation results; however the lunate remains aligned with the radius. Finally in stage IV, the lunate dislocates as a result of ulnotriquetral and dorsal radiocarpal tears. The lunate no longer remains within the lunate fossa and displaces volarly. The palmar ligaments which usually remain intact, cause the lunate to rotate into the carpal tunnel.

Herzberg[4] further classified the final lunate position in 1993. Stage I described a perilunate dislocation where the lunate remains in its place under the radius. A lunate that was palmarly displaced from the lunate fossa (perilunate dislocation with lunate dislocation) was categorized as stage II. Stage II lunate dislocations were further organized by the degree of rotation involved. A lunate rotated 90° was termed stage IIa, whereas stage IIb identified a lunate that was 180° rotated.

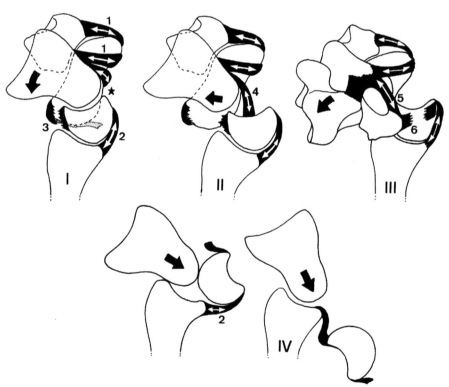

Fig. 2. Schematic of progressive perilunate instability. The characteristic sequence begins when the distal carpal row is forced into hyperextension (*dark arrows*). Stage I: the scapho-trapezoid-captiate ligaments (1) pull the scaphoid into extension opening up the space of Poirier (*asterisk*). The lunate, which is constrained by its volar ligaments (2), has a limited capacity to extend with the scaphoid before which the scapholunate ligament will fail (3). In stage II, the capitate dislocates dorsally from the lunate. The limit to dorsal translation is determined by the radioscaphoid-capitate ligament. In stage III, the energy propagates to the arcuate ligament (5), which pulls the triquetrum dorsally ultimately leading to a lunotriquetral ligament disruption (6). In stage IV, the lunate is pushed palmar in a rotatory fashion until it dislocates in to the carpal canal. (*From* Garcia-Elias M, Geissler WB Carpal instability. In: Green DP, Hotchkiss RN, Pederson WC, et al, eds. Green's Operative Hand Surgery, 5th ed Philadelphia; 2005. p. 535–604; with permission.)

Perilunate instability can occur through purely ligamentous means or in combination with fracture and are consequently subdivided into *perilunate dislocations* and *perilunate fracture dislocations*. *Lesser arc* injuries describe those that involve only ligamentous disruption. *Greater arc* injuries designate that a fracture of a bone or bones around the lunate has occurred. With greater arc injuries, the *trans* prefix is used to describe the fractured bones involved. Although Gilula originally described the normal arcs for radiographic interpretation in his classic article in 1979 (**Fig. 3**), Johnson[26] classified them into lesser arc and greater arc injuries. Recently, Bain and colleagues have modified Johnson's classification to describe a third pattern of injury termed *translunate arc*, which occurs through the lunate (**Fig. 4**).[27]

Common variants of perilunate injuries are trans-scaphoid or trans-styloid injuries. Uncommon variants include transtriquetral and transcapitate injuries. Scaphocapitate syndrome involves a particular dissipation of energy through the neck of the capitate. Other variants include scaphotrapezio-trapezoid dislocation that may replace the scapholunate dislocation or triquetro-hamate dislocation that may replace the lunotri-quetral dislocation within the perilunar instability model described by Mayfield.[1,28,29]

A reverse mechanism has been described contrary to Mayfield's radially initiated sequence of disruption. In a reverse Mayfield injury, reactive forces are directed toward the ulnar side of the wrist. Most often caused by a pronation-type injury, the pattern of sequential failure begins with the lunotriquetral ligament. The pathomechanics of ulnar-initiated perilunate instability has not been completely elucidated.[22,30–33]

DIAGNOSIS

Clinical and radiographic findings in perilunate injuries depend on the pattern of injury and multiple variations exist. Diagnosis requires a thorough history, complete physical examination, and appropriate imaging. Patients frequently describe a high-energy injury and present with a swollen, painful wrist. The carpus is most commonly dislocated dorsally, and physical examination reveals a prominent, palpable capitate. In acute injuries, soft tissue swelling may obscure bone landmarks. If the lunate is dislocated, it can encroach on the carpal tunnel and cause symptoms consistent with median nerve neuropathy. The incidence of acute carpal tunnel syndrome with perilunate injuries ranges from 16% to 46%.[34] Standard orthogonal views should be scrutinized for incongruity of arcs, intercarpal distance abnormalities, and disruption of angular associations between carpal bones (**Fig. 5**). Normal balance is assessed by the collinear alignment of the radius, lunate, capitate, and third metacarpal. Deviated values for the scapholunate angle (30–60°), radiolunate angle (<15°), and carpal height ratio (>0.5) provide objective evidence for injury. The posteroanterior (PA) view will demonstrate a loss of carpal arcs.[35] The scaphoid and lunate will fall into a flexed position and a cortical ring sign directs the clinician to consider a scapholunate ligament and/or lunotriquetral injury. The lunate will seem triangular and it will be displaced relative to the extent of energy imparted. Loss of articular alignment, overlap of carpal bones, and fractures may also be present. The lateral image will demonstrate alteration of the collinear alignment of the radius, lunate, and capitate.[36] The capitate is commonly displaced in a dorsal direction, and the lunate is displaced volarly. The lunate may be rotated 90° or 180°, resembling a spilled teacup.[36] A CT scan can delineate subtle fracture lines that may be present.

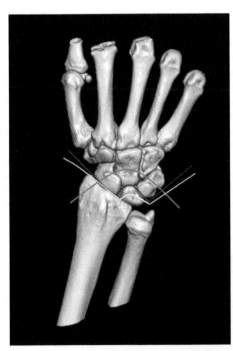

Fig. 3. CT image of the wrist demonstrating Bain's modification of Johnson's original classification of perilunate injury. The red line depicts a greater arc injury with fracture to the bones surrounding the lunate, which can include the radial styloid, scaphoid, capitate, hamate, and triquetrum. The blue line depicts a lesser arc injury representing disruption to the ligaments around the lunate. The yellow line describes a third pattern of injury, which occurs through the lunate.

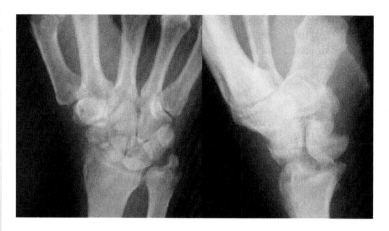

Fig. 4. Posteroanterior (PA) and lateral radiographic images of a trans-scaphoid perilunate dislocation. The PA view demonstrates a loss of carpal arcs and the lunate appears triangular. The lateral image demonstrates alteration of the collinear alignment of the radius, lunate, and capitate.

TREATMENT

The treatment of perilunate injuries has evolved over the years and includes closed reduction and immobilization,[37] closed reduction and percutaneous fixation,[38,39] external fixation combined with or without internal fixation,[40] open reduction and fixation with Kirschner wires (k wires) or screws,[4,41–45] lunate excision,[46] proximal row carpectomy,[47] and 4-corner fusion.[40]

Initial closed reduction maneuvers will relieve pressure on the median nerve and prevent further cartilage damage (**Fig. 6**). Traction for 10 to 15 minutes and analgesia may facilitate reduction. Closed reduction by itself is rarely a definitive treatment because the restoration of anatomy is critical to optimize the healing of ligaments and fractured bone. Adkison and Chapman[48] observed that 59% of the perilunate injuries that were anatomically realigned with closed reduction lost their reduction over time. It is not surprising, then, that closed reduction techniques combined with percutaneous pinning are not always successful in maintaining carpal alignment.[48]

Persistent carpal tunnel symptoms following closed reduction necessitates surgical intervention to release the transverse carpal ligament. Open injuries or the inability to achieve anatomic restoration following closed reduction are also indications for open treatment. If reduction is acceptable and median nerve symptoms are mild or nonprogressive, it is reasonable to perform delayed open reduction and fixation to ensure anatomic alignment. The authors know of no evidence that defines the time limits of when surgical treatment can be performed without compromising outcomes. Conventional wisdom, however, suggests that open reduction and internal fixation is best performed within the first several weeks following injury. A dorsal approach,[45] volar approach,[31] or combined dorsal and volar approach may be necessary and is often decided based on surgeon preference.[3,43,49–51]

The dorsal approach allows for easy visualization for carpal reduction, interosseous ligament repair, and fracture fixation. The volar approach allows decompression of the carpal tunnel and palmar capsule repair. Extensive volar dissection

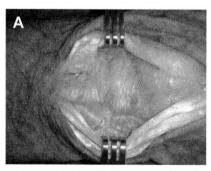
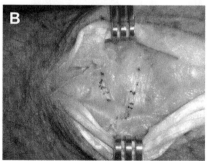

Fig. 5. The carpus is approached through a dorsal, longitudinal incision centered over the wrist. After the extensor pollicis longus is released, it is retracted radially while the extensor indicis proprius and extensor digitorum communis are retracted ulnarly (A). A radial-based dorsal ligament–sparing capsulotomy is performed according to that described by Berger in 1995[74] (depicted by blue dotted marker) (B).

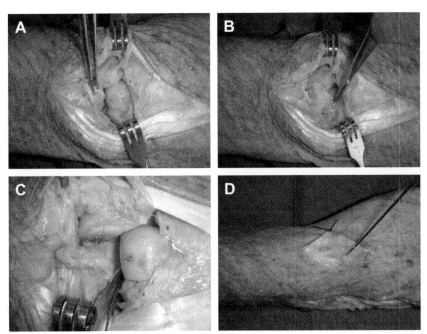

Fig. 6. After reduction of a perilunate dislocation, the capitate is frequently translated dorsally on the lunate and the scapholunate complex will still be dorsiflexed (*A*). Volar-directed pressure on neck of the capitate with a pair of forceps will drive the capitate in a more palmar location on the lunate and will rotate the scaphoid and lunate into a neutral position (*B*). Kirschner wires that were placed into the capitate and scaphoid prior to reduction are now advanced into the lunate to maintain carpal position. A counter incision is made over the radial aspect of the wrist to visualize and protect the radial sensory nerve.

should be avoided because Sotereanos and colleagues[49] reported a case of flexor tendon adhesions following combined volar approach with exploration and ligament repair. The technique for fixation is variable but involves some combination of k wires, headless compression screws, and lag screws. Trans-scaphoid fractures can be treated with[52] or without[43] bone graft from the distal radius; scaphoid comminution is a good indication for grafting. After open reduction and internal fixation of the scaphoid in trans-scaphoid perilunate dislocations, it is important to evaluate the integrity of the scapholunate and lunotriquetral ligament. Garcia-Elias and colleagues[53] found that trans-scaphoid patterns have a 3.8% incidence of concomitant complete scapholunate disruption. Stabilization with k-wire fixation has been described, but direct ligament repair and k-wire fixation seem to offer better maintenance of carpal alignment.[43,49,52] Repair is assumed to confer improved patient outcomes but this has not been objectively examined within the perilunate literature. K wires can be useful as joysticks to obtain adequate reduction of the scapholunate and lunotriquetral articulations. The scapholunate interosseous ligament often tears from the scaphoid and is repairable using braided polyester sutures. The lunotriquetral interosseous ligament is usually too injured for repair, and ligament augmentation may be necessary if serious injury is present. It is generally advised to reduce and repair the scapholunate ligament first followed by the lunotriquetral ligament. If primary repair cannot be performed, the authors suggest using a suture anchor. The extent of chondral injury should be documented during the procedure. Neurovascular checks should be performed as part of the preoperative and postoperative protocol. After surgery, patients are usually treated in a cast for 8 weeks and a splint for an additional 4 weeks. If k wires are used for fixation, they are typically removed at 12 weeks, although lunotriquetral k wires are commonly irritating and are usually removed earlier.

Recent popularity over arthroscopic-assisted percutaneous fixation for scaphoid fractures[54,55] has spurred the use of these alternative treatment options for trans-scaphoid perilunate dislocations.[56,57] Although results have demonstrated good functional outcomes in midterm follow-up (evidence of radiographic union, low morbidity/complication rate), the authors caution that larger series with matched controls and long-term follow-up will provide more information regarding the advantages and disadvantages of the technique before it is routinely used.[57]

Open reduction and internal fixation has become the treatment of choice for lesser and greater arc injuries.[4,34,38,45,49–52,58–64] The appropriate treatment of delayed injuries is, however, debated. In the past, it was considered inadvisable to attempt open reduction and internal fixation for injuries greater than 6 weeks out.[3,28] Proximal row carpectomy has been, for several years, the recommended salvage procedure for late presentation.[65] Newer evidence has suggested that this line of thinking is obsolete.

Kailu and colleagues[66] reported satisfactory results in their evaluation of 10 perilunate dislocations treated in a delayed fashion with open reduction and internal fixation (range: 3–6 weeks in the delayed group and 11–25 weeks in the chronic group). Patients were followed for an average of 90 months, and outcomes were based on the Cooney clinical scoring system and radiologic assessment. The average postoperative clinical scores were 81.0 (good) in the delayed group and 76.7 (good) in the chronic group. Scapholunate and radiolunate angles measured at early the postoperative follow-up and at the final follow-up remained in the range of the normal population in both groups according to the investigators. The mean range of motion and grip strength compared with the contralateral hand was $112 \pm 23°$ and 90% in the delayed group and $93 \pm 28°$ and 72% in the chronic group. The investigators note that cartilage condition of the midcarpal joint at the time of operation is critical to the treatment algorithm. If there is advanced wear, salvage procedures like proximal row carpectomy or arthrodesis should be considered.

AUTHORS' PREFERRED TREATMENT

On recognition of a perilunate injury, the wrist is inspected for signs of open wounds and an initial neurovascular examination is performed with particular attention to the median nerve. Closed reduction with sedation is attempted in the emergency department. If successful and patients have no median nerve symptoms, surgery is scheduled on an elective time frame, typically within a week's time. If the reduction is unsuccessful, patients are typically scheduled for surgical treatment within 24 hours. In the face of median nerve symptoms, open reduction and fixation of the carpus is accompanied by carpal tunnel release. A preoperative CT scan is obtained when a greater arc injury is present and when there is question about the extent of injury or alignment of the fracture carpus.

In the operating room, the authors prefer a regional block with sedation for anesthesia. Once the block seems effective, they attempt a second closed reduction of the wrist if the wrist was not relocated in the emergency department. It is the authors' experience that the tissue planes are less distorted following an effective reduction, making the surgical approach easier and safer. Fluoroscopic views are obtained to confirm adequate reduction. Adding a PA view with the wrist in ulnar deviation will help demonstrate associated radial styloid, scaphoid, capitate, hamate, and triquetral fractures.

The carpus is approached through a dorsal longitudinal incision centered over the wrist. The extensor pollicis longus is released from the third extensor compartment and retracted radially. The radial septum of the fourth compartment is released, and the extensor indicis proprius and extensor digitorum communis are retracted ulnarly. A Mayo dorsal ligament-sparing approach is used to gain access to the wrist (**Fig. 7**),[67] although the dorsal capsule may already be disrupted by the injury itself. If the carpus remains dislocated (typically the lunate), reduction is facilitated with a Freer elevator and manual traction to disengage and rotate the bones. The extent of

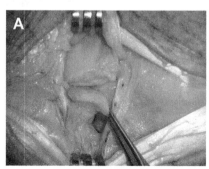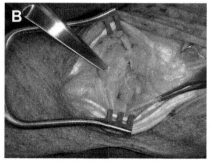

Fig. 7. The dorsal fibers of the scapholunate interosseous ligament often tear off its scaphoid attachment (*A*). It can be repaired primarily to bone using braided polyester sutures or suture anchors (*B*).

chondral injury is evaluated and documented. Note in particular the condition of the head of the capitate, often subject to shearing injuries when the head translates dorsally across the rim of the lunate (**Fig. 8**).

Fractures of the radial styloid are generally small fragments that the authors excise. Scaphoid fractures are reduced, held with a centrally placed pin from a cannulated screw set plus a second, parallel, antirotation pin placed dorsally and distally in scaphoid that avoids interference with screw placement. Permanent fixation consists of a headless screw supplemented with a distal radial bone graft for comminuted fractures. Fractures involving the head of the capitate are exposed with wrist flexion and held with 1 or 2 headless screws. Associated fractures of the triquetrum are usually volar and managed by reduction and pinning of the lunotriquetral joint. Fractures of the ulnar styloid are stabilized if there is instability of the distal radioulnar joint using pins and a tension band wiring technique or by using a small hook plate.

In lesser arc injuries, once the carpus is relocated, there will be residual rotation and diastasis present. The scaphoid will be pronated and flexed, the lunate extended, and the capitate flexed and translated posteriorly on the lunate. Two 0.045-in K wires are placed in a retrograde fashion through the scaphoid starting at its articulation with the lunate. When these pins exit the radial cortex of the scaphoid, a counterincision on the radial aspect of the wrist is useful to visualize and protect the radial sensory nerve. A third k wire is placed into the head of the capitate and advanced so that it exits in the zone between the radial wrist extensors and the finger extensors (**Fig. 9**). K wires are then placed in the dorsal cortex of the scaphoid and the lunate to use as joysticks. The scapholunate joint is reduced and held firmly with a small towel clip. The pins in the scaphoid are advanced into the lunate. At this juncture, the capitate will still

be translated dorsally on the lunate and the scapholunate complex will still be dorsiflexed. Volar-directed pressure on neck of the capitate with a pair of forceps will drive the capitate in a more palmer location on the lunate and will rotate the scaphoid and lunate into a neutral position. The pin in the capitate is then advanced into the lunate to maintain this position. The dorsal fibers of the scapholunate interosseous ligament often tear off its scaphoid attachment, whereas the lunotriquetral interosseous ligament is usually too injured for repair (**Fig. 10**). It is generally advised to repair the scapholunate ligament; if primary repair cannot be performed, the authors suggest using suture anchors. The lunotriquetral joint is reduced at this point and is held with one or two percutaneously placed pins. The scapholunate and capitolunate pins are bent and cut beneath the skin with care to place the cut pin tip away from adjacent tendon and nerves. The lunotriquetral pins are left outside of the skin or buried. Patients are immobilized in a splint for 2 weeks followed by a short arm and thumb spica cast for 2 weeks. The authors encourage immediate finger motion and forearm rotation. At 4 weeks, the exposed lunotriquetral pins are removed and a cast is reapplied. At 8 weeks, patients are transitioned to a wrist splint and permitted intermittent active wrist motion out of the splint. At 12 weeks, the remaining pins are removed and the authors prescribe formal therapy. At every juncture, patients are counseled about residual median nerve symptoms, wrist stiffness, and the possibility of posttraumatic arthritis, particularly of the midcarpal joint.

COMPLICATIONS

Complications following perilunate injury include median nerve neuropathy, chondrolysis, residual carpal instability, complex regional pain syndrome, attritional rupture of tendons, wrist stiffness, posttraumatic arthritis, and compromised

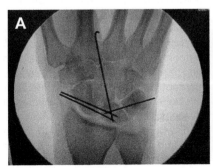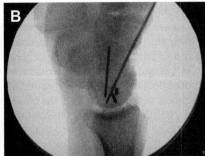

Fig. 8. PA (A) and lateral (B) images demonstrating the appropriate position of intercarpal pins after reduction and ligamentous stabilization of a perilunate dislocation.

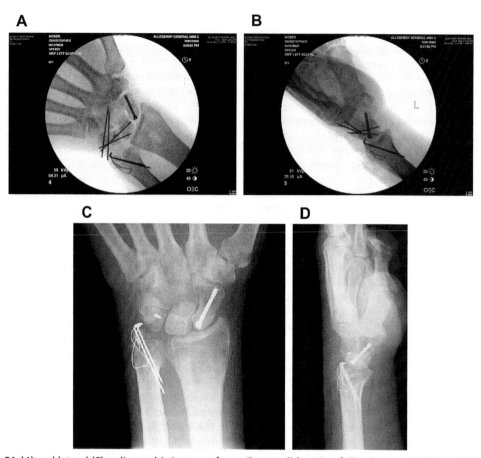

Fig. 9. PA (*A*) and lateral (*B*) radiographic images of a perilunate dislocation following repair. The scaphoid frac ture was treated with cannulated screw fixation and the lunotriquetral ligament was repaired with the aid of a suture anchor. The lunotriquetral and triquetro-capitate intervals were pinned with 0.045-in Kirschner wires to hold an adequate reduction, and the ulnar styloid was fixed using tension band technique. Ten months following repair, the patient had functional range of motion. Two-year radiographic follow-up demonstrates preserved carpal alignment (*C and D*).

hand function. In Herzberg and colleagues'[4] series, acute carpal tunnel syndrome accompanied 23% of the injuries.[4] The incidence in the current litera- ture ranges from 16% to 46%.[34] Transient ischemia, identified radiographically by increased density of the lunate, should not be confused with avascular necrosis of the lunate because the blood supply to the lunate is preserved. Transient ischemia of the lunate can last several months; however, it is a self-limiting disorder.[68] Chondroly- sis can occur at the radiocarpal and midcarpal joint; it predisposes to early progressive arthritis and is most commonly seen at the head of the capi- tate. Persistent carpal instability, frequently observed at the scapholunate, lunotriquetral, or midcarpal joint, and fracture malunion and nonunion are increased when fracture dislocations are treated by closed means.

OUTCOMES

Results depend on the severity of the initial injury, accurate and timely diagnosis, and the quality of the reduction. Successful outcomes are inversely related to delay in treatment, open injury, chondral damage, instability, and malunion. Open anatomic repair seems to provide the clinician with a better chance of a favorable outcome.[4,51,59] Most outcome studies focus on range of motion, pain, and grip strength,[4,45,51,52,69] although patient perception by validated measures is limited.[60,61,70]

Cooney retrospectively evaluated 30 perilunate dislocations; 9 were treated with cast immobiliza- tion, whereas 21 were treated with open reduc- tion and internal fixation.[69] Twenty-eight out of 30 were followed an average of 3 years after treatment and 15 out of 30 were available for long-term follow-up (greater than 5 years). Pain,

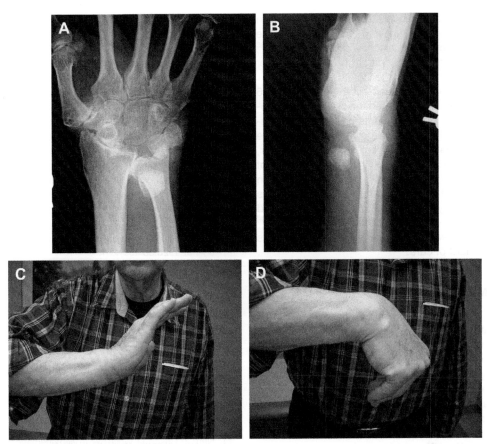

Fig. 10. PA (*A*) and lateral (*B*) images of a lunate dislocation identified 10 months following injury. The patient had remarkable range of motion and little residual pain (*C and D*). Unfortunately, these results are atypical; early and appropriate recognition of these injuries can avoid debilitating outcomes.

functional status, range of motion, and grip strength were used to derive a clinical rating using a modified rating system by Green and O'Brien.[3] Based on the results, the authors advocated open reduction and fixation in the setting of scaphoid fractures that were malaligned, had scapholunate instability, persistent lunate instability, or injuries with the presence of trans-scaphoid or transcapitate fractures. Relatively stable fracture dislocations could be treated with immobilization; however, persistent instability and loss of reduction was a problem in this cohort of patients.

Kremer and colleagues[70] retrospectively evaluated 39 patients with perilunate injuries (with 30 out of 39 involving fractures) treated with open reduction, ligament reconstruction, and/or internal fixation. At a mean follow-up of 65.5 months, the investigators found satisfactory results; however, loss of motion and grip strength was significant. Visual analog scale pain scores were 1.8 at rest and 4.8 with activities. Grip strength was 36.6 kg

(vs 51.6 kg in contralateral limb), and arc of wrist range of motion was 77°. MAYO wrist scores (70) and Disabilities of the Arm, Shoulder, and Hand scores (23) were thought to be acceptable considering the magnitude of injury in most cases. On final follow-up, 20 out of 39 patients had evidence of radiocarpal arthrosis, 18 had increased scapholunate angles, and 6 patients had ulnar shifting at the carpus. The investigators mention that outcomes seem to worsen over time in contrast to studies with shorter-term follow-up.[59,62]

Perilunate injuries are associated with a high incidence of posttraumatic arthrosis. The current literature notes the mean incidence as 38%, with a range from 7% to 92%.[4,45,71,72] Forli and colleagues[73] retrospectively reviewed 18 patients with perilunate dislocations (11) and trans-scaphoid perilunate fracture dislocations (7), all treated with open reduction internal fixation at a minimum follow-up of 10 years. Posttraumatic degenerative changes were observed in 12 out of 18 cases (68%), but they were not associated with reduced function. This finding follows previously reported studies with medium-term follow-up and suggests that the radiographic-exhibited arthritis is well tolerated.[45] The rate of degenerative change, however, is higher than previous reports in the literature.[4,45,59,61]

Herzberg and colleagues,[4] in their series of 166 perilunate injuries, evaluated the clinical and radiologic outcome of 115 patients and found that delayed treatment was associated with adverse clinical effects. Kailu and colleagues,[66] however, found satisfactory results in the evaluation of 10 perilunate dislocations treated with open reduction and internal fixation at least 3 weeks following injury (range: 3–6 weeks in the delayed group and 11–25 weeks in the chronic group).[66] Early open treatment is still largely advocated as the standard of care.

SUMMARY

The progressive perilunar instability model described by Mayfield and colleagues[1] is still used today to predict the pattern of injury. Multiple variations of the same injury pattern exist depending on energy propagation. Injuries can involve bone or simple ligament disruption. Diagnosis of injury and clinical and radiographic findings depend on the pattern of injury present. Open procedures are preferred for anatomic reduction after initial closed reduction is performed for acute injuries. A dorsal approach,[45] volar approach,[31] or a combined dorsal and volar approach[49] may be necessary and is often decided by surgeon preference. Results largely depend on the severity of the initial injury, accurate and timely diagnosis, and quality of reduction. Unfortunately, loss of motion and diminished grip strength are common consequences despite appropriate treatment. Successful outcomes depend on time to treatment, open or closed nature of the injury, extent of chondral damage, residual instability, and fracture union. Although post-traumatic arthrosis is common, it is not associated with diminished function after midterm and long-term follow-up, suggesting that the radiographic exhibited arthritis is well tolerated.[45,73]

REFERENCES

1. Mayfield JK, Johnson RP, Kilcoyne RK. Carpal dislocations: pathomechanics and progressive perilunar instability. J Hand Surg Am 1980;5(3):226–41.
2. Fenton RL. The naviculo-capitate fracture syndrome. J Bone Joint Surg Am 1956;38(3):681–4.
3. Green DP, O'Brien ET. Open reduction of carpal dislocations: indications and operative techniques. J Hand Surg Am 1978;3(3):250–65.
4. Herzberg G, Comtet JJ, Linscheid RL, et al. Perilunate dislocations and fracture-dislocations: a multicenter study. J Hand Surg Am 1993;18:768–79.
5. Siegert JJ, Frassica FJ, Amadio PC. Treatment of chronic perilunate dislocations. J Hand Surg Am 1988;13:206–12.
6. Ruby LK, Cooney WP, An KN, et al. Relative motion of selected carpal bones: a kinematic analysis of the normal wrist. J Hand Surg 1988;13(1):1–10.
7. Bryce TH. Certain points in the anatomy and mechanism of the wrist-joint reviewed in the light of a series of Rontgen Ray photographs of the living hand. J Anat Physiol 1896;31:59–79.
8. Von Bonin G. A note on the kinematics of the wrist joint. J Anat 1919;63:259–62.
9. Cyriax EF. On the rotary movements of the wrist. J Anat 1926;60:199–201.
10. Wright RD. A detailed study of movement of the wrist joint. J Anat 1935;70:137–42.
11. Arkless R. Cineradiography in normal and abnormal wrists. Am J Roentgenol Radium Ther Nucl Med 1966;96(4):837–44.
12. Erdman AG, Mayfield JK, Dorman F, et al. Kinematic and kinetic analysis of the human wrist by stereoscopic instrumentation. J Biomech Eng 1979;101:124–33.
13. Berger RA, Crowninshield RD, Flatt AE. The three-dimensional rotational behaviors of the carpal bones. Clin Orthop Relat Res 1982;167:303–10.
14. Neu CP, Crisco JJ, Wolfe SW. In vivo kinematic behavior of the radio-capitate joint during wrist flexion-extension and radio-ulnar deviation. J Biomech 2001;34(11):1429–38.
15. Navarro A. Anales de instituto de clinica quirurgica y cirugia experimental. Montevideo (MN): Imprenta Artistica de Dornaleche Hnos; 1935.
16. Taleisnik J. Current concepts review. Carpal instability. J Bone Joint Surg Am 1988;70:1262–8.
17. Weber ER. Concepts governing the rotational shift of the intercalated segment of the carpus. Orthop Clin North Am 1984;15(2):193–207.
18. deLange A, Kauer JM, Huiskes R. Kinematic behavior of the human wrist joint: a roentgen-stereophotogrammetric analysis. J Orthop Res 1985;3:56–64.
19. Linscheid JH, Dobyns JH, Beabout JW, et al. Traumatic instability of the wrist. J Bone Joint Surg Am 1972;54(8):1612–32.
20. Linscheid RL, Dobyns JH. Carpal instability. Curr Orthop 1989;3:106–14.
21. Gilford WW, Bolton RH, Lambrinudi C. The mechanism of the wrist joint with special reference to fractures of the scaphoid. Guys Hospital Reports 1943;92:52–9.
22. Lichtman DM, Schneider JR, Swafford AR, et al. Ulnar midcarpal instability: clinical and laboratory analysis. J Hand Surg 1981;6(5):515–23.

23. Linscheid RL. Kinematic considerations of the wrist. Clin Orthop Relat Res 1986;24(2):164–8.

24. Lichtman DM, Bruckner JD, Culp RW, et al. Palmar midcarpal instability: results of surgical reconstruction. J Hand Surg 1993;18(2):307–15.

25. Amadio PC. Carpal Kinematics and instability: a clinical and anatomic primer. Clin Anat 1991;4(1):1–12.

26. Johnson RP. The acutely injured wrist and its residuals. Clin Orthop Relat Res 1980;149:33–44.

27. Bain GI, McLean JM, Turner PC, et al. Translunate fracture with associated perilunate injury: 3 case reports with introduction of the translunate arc concept. J Hand Surg 2008;33(10):1770–6.

28. Fisk GR. The wrist. J Bone Joint Surg Br 1984;66(3):396–407.

29. Bohler L. The treatment of fractures. 5th edition. New York: Grune & Stratton, Inc; 1965. p. 854–81.

30. Trumble TE, Bour CJ, Smith RJ, et al. Kinematics of the ulnar carpus related to the volar intercalated segment instability pattern. J Hand Surg 1990; 15(3):384–92.

31. Viegas SF, Patterson RM, Peterson PD, et al. Ulnar-sided perilunate instability: an anatomic and biomechanic study. J Hand Surg Am 1990;15(2):266–78.

32. Dobyns JH, Linscheid RL, Macksoud WS. Carpal instability nondissociative. J Hand Surg Br 1994; 19:763–73.

33. Horii E, Garcia-Elias M, An KN, et al. A kinematic study of luno-triquetral dissociations. J Hand Surg Am 1991;16(2):334–9.

34. Trumble T, Verheyden J. Treatment of isolated perilunate and lunate dislocations with combined dorsal and volar approach and intraosseous cerclage wire. J Hand Surg Am 2004;29(3):412–7.

35. Gilula LA. Carpal injuries: analytic approach and case exercises. AJR Am J Roentgenol 1979; 133(3):503–17.

36. Green DP, O'Brien ET. Classification and management of carpal dislocations. Clin Orthop Relat Res 1980;149:55–72.

37. Russell TB. Inter-carpal dislocations and fracture-dislocations; a review of 59 cases. J Bone Joint Surg Br 1949;31(4):524–31.

38. Komurcu M, Kurklu M, Ozturan KE, et al. Early and delayed treatment of dorsal transscaphoid perilunate fracture-dislocations. J Orthop Trauma 2008; 22(8):535–40.

39. Slade JF, Gutow AP, Geissler WB. Percutaneous internal fixation of scaphoid fractures via an arthroscopically assisted dorsal approach. J Bone Joint Surg Am 2002;84(Suppl 2):21–36.

40. Wagner CJ. Perilunar dislocations. J Bone Joint Surg Am 1956;38(6):1198–207.

41. Hee HT, Wong HP, Low YP. Transscaphoid perilunate fracture/dislocations – results of surgical treatment. Ann Acad Med Singapore 1999;28(6):791–4.

42. Viegas SF, Bean JW, Schram RA. Transscaphoid fracture/dislocations treated with open reduction and Herbert screw internal fixation. J Hand Surg Am 1987;12(6):992–9.

43. Moneim MS, Hofammann KE, Omer GE. Transscaphoid perilunate fracture-dislocation. Result of open reduction and pin fixation. Clin Orthop Relat Res 1984;190:227–35.

44. DiGiovanni B, Shaffer J. Treatment of perilunate and transscaphoid perilunate dislocations of the wrist. Am J Orthop 1995;24(11):818–26.

45. Herzberg G, Forissier D. Acute dorsal trans-scaphoid perilunate fracture-dislocations: medium-term results. J Hand Surg Br 2002;27(6):498–502.

46. MacAusland WR. Perilunar dislocation of the carpal bones and dislocation of the lunate bone. Surg Gynecol Obstet 1944;79:256.

47. Campbell RD, Thompson TC, Lance EM, et al. Indications for open reduction of lunate and perilunate dislocations of the carpal bones. J Bone Joint Surg Am 1965;49:915–37.

48. Adkison JW, Chapman MW. Treatment of acute lunate and perilunate dislocations. Clin Orthop Relat Res 1982;164:199–207.

49. Sotereanos DG, Mitsionis GJ, Giannakopoulos PN, et al. Perilunate dislocation and fracture dislocation: a critical analysis of the volar-dorsal approach. J Hand Surg Am 1997;22(1):49–56.

50. Inoue G, Imaeda T. Management of trans-scaphoid perilunate dislocations. Herbert screw fixation, ligamentous repair and early wrist mobilization. Arch Orthop Trauma Surg 1997;116(6–7):338–40.

51. Apergis E, Maris J, Theodoratos G, et al. Perilunate dislocations and fracture-dislocations. Closed and early open reduction compared in 28 cases. Acta Orthop Scand Suppl 1997;275:55–9.

52. Knoll VD, Allan C, Trumble TE. Trans-scaphoid perilunate fracture dislocations: results of screw fixation of the scaphoid and lunotriquetral repair with a dorsal approach. J Hand Surg Am 2005;30(6):1145–52.

53. Garcia-Elias M, Ribe M, Rodriguez J, et al. Influence of joint laxity on scaphoid kinematics. J Hand Surg Br 1995;20(3):379–82.

54. Weil WM, Slad JF, Trumble TE. Open and arthroscopic treatment of perilunate injuries. Clin Orthop Relat Res 2006;445:120–32.

55. Wong TC, Ip FK. Minimally invasive management of trans-scaphoid perilunate fracture-dislocations. Hand Surg 2008;13(3):159–65.

56. Park MJ, Ahn JH. Arthroscopically assisted reduction and percutaneous fixation of dorsal perilunate dislocations and fracture-dislocations. Arthroscopy 2005;21(9):1153.

57. Jeon IH, Kim HJ, Min WK, et al. Arthroscopically assisted percutaneous fixation for trans-scaphoid perilunate fracture dislocation. J Hand Surg Eur Vol 2010;35(8):664–8.

58. Perron AD, Brady WJ, Keats TE, et al. Orthopedic pitfalls in the ED: scaphoid fracture. Am J Emerg Med 2001;19(4):310–6.

59. Inoue G, Kuwahata Y. Management of acute perilunate dislocations without fracture of the scaphoid. J Hand Surg Br 1997;22(5):647–52.

60. Souer JS, Rutgers M, Andermahr J, et al. Perilunate fracture-dislocations of the wrist: comparison of temporary screw versus K-wire fixation. J Hand Surg Am 2007;32(3):318–25.

61. Hildebrand KA, Ross DC, Patterson SD, et al. Dorsal perilunate dislocations and fracture-dislocations: questionnaire, clinical, and radiographic evaluation. J Hand Surg Am 2000;25(6):1069–79.

62. Inoue G, Tanaka Y, Nakamura R. Treatment of trans-scaphoid perilunate dislocations by internal fixation with the Herbert screw. J Hand Surg Br 1990;15(4):449–54.

63. Minami A, Kaneda K. Repair and/or reconstruction of scapholunate interosseous ligament in lunate and perilunate dislocations. J Hand Surg Am 1993; 18(6):1099–106.

64. Inoue G, Shionoya K. Late treatment of unreduced perilunate dislocations. J Hand Surg 1999;24(2):221–5.

65. Campbell RD, Lance EM, Yeow CB. Lunate and perilunar dislocations. J Bone Joint Surg Br 1964; 46:55–72.

66. Kailu L, Zhou X, Fuguo H. Chronic perilunate dislocations treated with open reduction and internal fixation: results of medium-term follow-up. Int Orthop 2010;34(8):1315–20.

67. Berger RA. A method of defining palpable landmarks for the ligament-splitting dorsal wrist capsulotomy. J Hand Surg Am 2007;32:1291–5.

68. White RE, Omer GE. Transient vascular compromise of the lunate after fracture-dislocation of dislocation of the carpus. J Hand Surg Am 1984;9:181–4.

69. Cooney WP, Bussey R, Dobyns JH, et al. Difficult wrist fractures. Perilunate fracture-dislocations of the wrist. Clin Orthop Relat Res 1987;214:136–47.

70. Kremer T, Wendt M, Riedel K, et al. Open reduction for perilunate injuries – clinical outcome and patient satisfaction. J Hand Surg Am 2010;35(10):1599–606.

71. Altissimi M, Mancini GB, Assara A. Perilunate dislocations of the carpus. A long-term review. Ital J Orthop Traumatol 1987;13(4):491–500.

72. Pai CH, Wei DC, Hu ST. Carpal bone dislocations: an analysis of twenty cases with relative emphasis on the role of crushing mechanisms. J Trauma 1993; 35(1):28–35.

73. Forli A, Courvoisier A, Wimsey S, et al. Perilunate dislocations and transscaphoid perilunate fracture dislocations: a retrospective study with minimum ten-year follow-up. J Hand Surg Am 2010;35(1):62–8.

74. Berger RA, Bishop AT, Bettinger PC. New dorsal capsulotomy for the surgical exposure of the wrist. Ann Plast Surg 1995;35(1):54–9.

The Scaphoid

Rosie Sendher, MD, MHSC, Amy L. Ladd, MD*

KEYWORDS

• Scaphoid • Wrist function • Carpal fractures • Distal radius • Upper extremity trauma

KEY POINTS

- Almost completely covered with articular cartilage, this creates precise surface loading demands and intolerance to bony remodeling.
- Fracture location compounds risk of malunion and nonunion.
- Scaphoid fractures may significantly impair wrist function and activities of daily living, with both individual and economic consequences.

INTRODUCTION

The scaphoid is vitally important for proper mechanics of wrist function. Its unique morphology from its boat-like shape to its retrograde blood supply can present with challenges in the presence of a fracture. Almost completely covered with articular cartilage, this creates precise surface loading demands and intolerance to bony remodeling. Fracture location compounds risk of malunion and nonunion. Scaphoid fractures may significantly impair wrist function and activities of daily living, with both individual and economic consequences.

Epidemiology

The scaphoid is the most commonly fractured carpal bone, accounting for approximately 70% of carpal fractures, and the second most common fracture of the upper extremity after distal radius fractures. The majority occurs from a low-energy injury, such as a fall onto an outstretched wrist from standing height. High-energy mechanisms such as a fall from a height or motor vehicle injury account for the remainder.

The highest incidence of fractures occur in younger age groups; 1 study found the highest incidence in males between the ages of 20 and 29 years old.[1,2] Similarly, a Norwegian study found an average age of male individuals with scaphoid fractures to be 25 years old. Wolf recently studied the US military population and found an incidence of scaphoid fractures to be 121 per 100,000 person-years.[3] The higher incidence was in males in the 20- to 24-year age group is likely owing to the more active nature of the military population. Wolf's study using a public database of acute injuries with the US general population, found that there is a male predominance of 66.4%, and thus the remaining 33.6% female representing a higher incidence than the typically reported in the previous studies.[3] They postulated that the increased incidence in females over the years were likely owing to an increased participation in organized sports.

Anatomy

The scaphoid has an unusual shape; the name is derived from the Greek word "skaphe" for 'boat.' The early 20th century nomenclature used 'navicular,' Latin for 'boat.' Given its odd and complex configuration, defining the exact fracture pattern or degree of displacement can be problematic. It appears concave in both ulnar and palmar axes. Its long axis is on an oblique plane. It is the largest bone in the proximal carpal row.

Four different regions of the scaphoid have been described. They are the tubercle, waist, distal

Department of Orthopaedic Surgery, Stanford School of Medicine, 450 Broadway Street, Pavilion A, Redwood City, CA 94063, USA
* Corresponding author.
E-mail address: alad@stanford.edu

Orthop Clin N Am 44 (2013) 107–120
http://dx.doi.org/10.1016/j.ocl.2012.09.003
0030-5898/13/$ – see front matter © 2013 Elsevier Inc. All rights reserved.

pole, and proximal pole. The scaphoid is 75% articular, especially the ulnar side. Proximally, the scaphoid articulates with the distal radius at the scaphoid fossa, and distally with the trapezoid and trapezium. Ulnarly, it articulates with the lunate proximally and the capitate distally. The volar surface is partly nonarticular. The tubercle, which points radiovolarly, serves as an attachment for several ligaments and is also almost entirely covered by the crossing flexor carpi radialis (FCR) tendon. The scaphoid is oriented in the carpus with an intrascaphoid angle averaging approximately 40° in the coronal plane and 30° in the sagittal plane. Heinzelmann and colleagues[4] found that male scaphoids were significantly longer (by 4 mm) and wider in their proximal pole than female scaphoids. The implications for surgical screw sizing based on sex and habitus often leads to recommending smaller screw sizes for female patients when considering operative fixation.[5]

The majority of scaphoid fractures occur at the waist, and this higher incidence may also be related to the structural properties of the bone. Bindra[6] studied cadaveric scaphoid with computed tomography (CT) and found that the bone is most dense at the proximal pole, where the trabeculae are the thickest and are more tightly packed, whereas the trabeculae in the waist are thinnest and sparsely distributed.

The dorsoradial ridge separates the dorsal and proximal articular surfaces from the distal volar aspect. The ridge is a narrow and nonarticulating area with several vascular perforations allowing important perfusion of the scaphoid. About 70 to 80% of the intraosseous vascularity and the entire proximal pole are supplied from branches of the radial artery entering through this ridge. Having a singular dominant intraosseous vessel predisposes the scaphoid to avascular necrosis (AVN)[7–12] and nonunion if fractured. With the predominantly articular nature of the scaphoid, there are few potential sites for the entrance of perforating vessels; thus, it has a tenuous vascular supply. The major palmar blood vessels arise from either the radial artery directly or the superficial palmar arch and divide into several smaller branches before coursing obliquely and distally over the palmar aspect of the scaphoid to enter through the region of the tubercle. The anterior interosseus artery provides collateral circulation to the scaphoid. In addition, Herbert and Lanzetta have hypothesized that there must be some blood supply through the scapholunate ligament complex.[13] From their cases series, proximal pole fragments remained viable when their only remaining attachment was to the SLIL.

Given the predominantly articular surface of the scaphoid, its attached ligaments play a critical role in stability and mechanics of the wrist. The scaphoid links the proximal and distal carpal rows, and as such influences motion at each row depending its position and functional demand.[7,13–15] The scapholunate ligament is intra-articular and connects the scaphoid and lunate at the proximal aspect of their articulation with 3 main parts. The dorsal aspect of the ligament is the strongest and thickest, and composed of transverse collagen fibers. The dorsal portion is twice as strong as the palmar portion. The dorsal region resists palmar-dorsal translation and gap. The volar portion is not as strong as the dorsal portion, and the proximal or membranous portion is made of fibrocartilage and is not truly a ligament.

The radioscaphocapitate (RSC) ligament originates from the radial styloid and lies in the volar concavity of the scaphoid waist. It attaches the capitate ulnarly. The RSC acts as fulcrum to allow scaphoid rotation. It may also have a proprioceptive role, because it contains a high density of mechanoreceptors. The scaphocapitate ligament originates from the distal scaphoid. It inserts into the volar waist of the capitate distal to the RSC ligament. This ligament, along with the scaphotrapezial ligament, functions as a primary restraint of the distal pole.[13]

With displaced scaphoid fractures, the proximal pole extends because of its attachment to the lunate through the scapholunate ligament, whereas the distal fragment remains flexed because of its attachment to the trapezium and trapezoid via the scaphotrapezial ligament. These deforming forces lead to a humpback deformity. The anatomy of the scaphoid and its associated ligaments contribute greatly to the risk of malunion and nonunion. It is almost completely covered with articular cartilage, limiting the amount of surface area for bone contact and healing. Displacement of these articular fracture fragments can also allow synovial fluid to pass between them and delay or halt healing.

KINEMATICS

Carpal kinematic studies provide several theories indicating a bone in a given carpal row (proximal or distal) will move in the same direction with varying magnitudes.[14,15] Wolfe and colleagues[15] challenged that wrist motion cannot be readily simplified into a 2-linkage system. In their study they used a 3-dimensional CT technique to study carpal kinematics. They found significant intercarpal motion between the scaphoid and lunate that negate a 2 linkage system explaining wrist kinematics. Wolfe and colleagues[15] further postulated that the scaphoid should be regarded as independent from the carpal rows and that its kinematics are determined by direction and magnitude of wrist motion and its neighboring bones. They studied uninjured wrists with a markerless bone registration technique using 3-dimensional CT and confirmed that the amount of rotation of each of these bones depends on the direction of the wrist motion. The scaphoid extends with ulnar deviation and flexes with radial deviation. There is a neutral position when the scaphoid flexion and extension occurs between 10° and 15° off of the sagittal plane along the dart thrower's path. In this plane of motion, there is a transition between the scaphoid and lunate flexion and extension whereby motions of the 2 bones were minimal.

Classification

In general, scaphoid waist fractures are the most common at 70%, distal pole fractures compromise 10%–20%, proximal pole fractures are 5%, and tubercle fractures make up 5%. Herbert classified fractures in to stable acute, unstable acute, delayed union, and nonunion. Russe classified scaphoid fractures into horizontal oblique, transverse, or vertical oblique patterns (**Fig. 1**). The Herbert classification attempts to define stable and unstable fractures and therefore may be particularly helpful in determining treatment options. The type A Herbert classification fracture is a stable acute fracture and type B is an unstable acute fracture. Stable fractures include fractures of the tubercle (A1) and an incomplete fracture of the

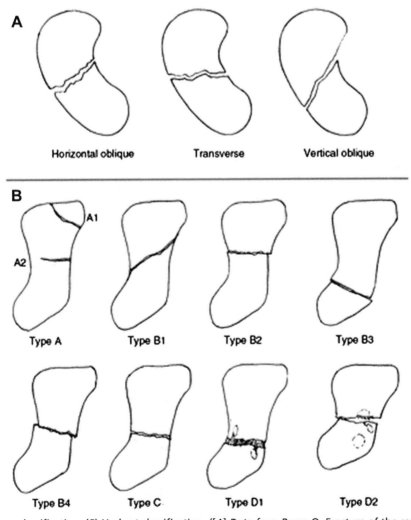

Fig. 1. (*A*) Russe classification. (*B*) Herbert classification. ([*A*] *Data from* Russe O. Fracture of the carpal navicular: diagnosis, non-operative treatment, and operative treatment. J Bone Joint Surg Am 1960;42:759–68; and [*B*] *Data from* Herbert TJ. The fractured scaphoid. St. Louis (MO): Quality Medical Publishing; 1990.)

waist (A2). These fractures can potentially be treated nonoperatively. The other types of fractures in the Herbert classification usually require operative treatment. Type B fractures (acute unstable fractures) include subtypes B1 (oblique fractures of the distal third), B2 (displaced or mobile fractures of the waist), B3 (proximal pole fractures), B4 (fracture dislocations), and B5 (comminuted fractures). Type C fractures show delayed union after more than 6 weeks of plaster immobilization, whereas type D fractures are established nonunions, either fibrous (D1) or sclerotic (D2).

ACUTE SCAPHOID FRACTURE
Presentation

The mechanism of injury is typically a fall onto an outstretched hand with the wrist in an extended position, placing the scaphoid vertical and making it vulnerable to injury. Patients may complain of vague or dorsal wrist pain, weakness, and limitation with range of motion, especially with flexion and radial deviation. On physical examination,

tenderness may be present with palpation at the anatomic snuffbox, the distal scaphoid tubercle, and at the proximal pole dorsally. Longitudinal compression of the thumb may also elicit symptoms. Other findings may include crepitus, instability, swelling—including loss of the concavity of anatomic snuffbox—and ecchymosis.

Standard posterioanterior, lateral, and oblique radiographs (45°–60° of pronation) should be obtained (**Fig. 2**). Scaphoid views are particularly helpful to visualize the scaphoid architecture and look for fractures. Special views such as clenched fist views can be useful to rule out suspected scapholunate injury if no fracture is readily identified and clinical suspicion is high. The intra-scaphoid angle is the intersection of 2 lines drawn perpendicular to the diameters of the proximal and distal poles. Normal is less than 35°. An angle greater than 35° suggests a humpback deformity. The height/length ratio of the scaphoid is used to indicate collapse. Normal values are greater than 0.65.

If the radiographs are negative initially, patients may be treated with cast immobilization in a thumb spica splint for 2 weeks before re-imaging. These

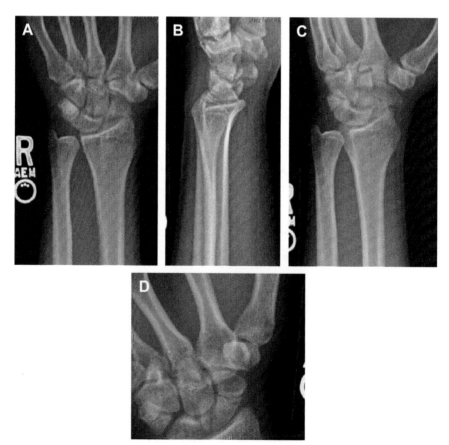

Fig. 2. (A–D) Posterioanterior, lateral, oblique, and scaphoid views. The scaphoid view demonstrates a waist fracture.

ollow-up x-rays may show bone resorption adjacent to the fracture site, thus making the nondisplaced fracture visible. If the initial x-rays readily identify a scaphoid fracture, this may represent displacement[16] and acute operative treatment is indicated.

Other radiographic modalities can make rapid diagnoses and prevent unnecessary immobilization in those patients with suspected, but not true fractures. Although no longer commonplace for identification of scaphoid fractures, bone scans show increased uptake in the area of the scaphoid within 24 hours (**Fig. 3**). A focal increased activity correlated with a clinical examination indicates an acute fracture. CT allows for an accurate analysis of the bony anatomy, allows fracture pattern characterization, and can be used for surgical planning.[16] The sagittal cuts, along the axis of the scaphoid, are best to define any collapse or humpback deformity at the fracture site (**Fig. 4**). The lateral intrascaphoid angle and height to length ratio can be measured. CT can also be used to follow healing, as a better assessment can be made of any cortical bridging.

The average sensitivity of CT for a nondisplaced fracture is 89% and specificity is 91%.[16] CT should be used with caution for triage of nondisplaced scaphoid fractures because false-positive results occur, perhaps from misinterpretation of vascular foraminae or other normal lines in the scaphoid. Given the relative infrequency of true fractures among patients with suspected scaphoid fractures, CT is better for ruling out a fracture than for ruling one in.

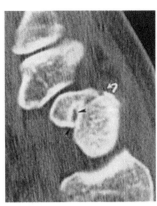

Fig. 4. CT and arrow demonstrating a humpback deformity. (*From* Yin YM, McEnery KW, Gilula LA. Computed tomography. In: Gilula LA, Yin YM, editors. Imaging of the wrist and hand. Philadelphia: Saunders; 1996. p. 425.)

Magnetic resonance imaging (MRI) is more sensitive and specific to detect an occult fracture.[16] One can also assess both the osseous blood supply and soft tissue integrity. Studies have been done to compare the cost of an initial MRI versus serial radiographic evaluation. Brooks and colleagues[17] performed a randomized, controlled trial investigated the cost-effectiveness of MRI for diagnosing suspected scaphoid fractures. There were 28 patients enrolled who had a suspected scaphoid fracture. Patients were randomized to undergo MRI scan or conservative treatment with immobilization and serial clinical and radiographic evaluation. Those who underwent MRI had a shorter duration of immobilization and decreased use of health care resources but increased cost to treat compared with patients randomized to the non-MRI group, who were immobilized and evaluated with serial clinical and radiographic examination. Cost per day of unnecessary immobilization between the groups was $44.37. The costs did not include work absence. Another study by Pillai and Jain[18] reported a rate of more than 80% of unnecessary immobilization for suspected scaphoid fractures and negative radiographs. They concluded that the cost of needless immobilization, with further clinical and radiographic studies, would have exceeded early alternative investigations, such as MRI or bone scan, which were frequently required anyway.[16] An MRI is also very useful in suspected cases of AVN with respect to diagnosis and surgical planning (**Fig. 5**).

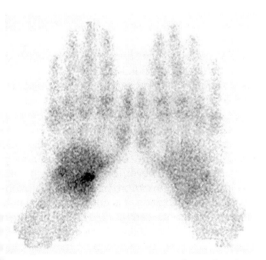

Fig. 3. Bone scan showing increased uptake. (*Data from* van Vugt RM, Bijlsma JW, van Vugt AC. Chronic wrist pain: diagnosis and management. Development and use of a new algorithm. Ann Rheum Dis 1999; 58:665–74. http://dx.doi.org/10.1136/ard.58.11.665.)

Nonoperative Treatment

Distal or tubercle fractures often heal adequately with cast immobilization. Nonoperative treatment

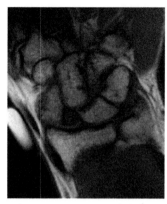

Fig. 5. MRI demonstrating AVN of the scaphoid. Outcome after vascularized bone grafting of scaphoid nonunions with avascular necrosis. (*From* Waitayawinyu T, McCallister WV, Katolik LI, et al. Outcome after vascularized bone grafting of scaphoid nonunions with avascular necrosis. J Hand Surg Am 2009;34(3):387–94; with permission.)

involves a long-arm or short-arm thumb spica cast, with the wrist in neutral position leaving the thumb interphalangeal joint free. This cast is maintained for 8 weeks and then CT can be done to assess healing. If the CT still suggests unhealed fracture, cast immobilization is maintained for another 4 to 6 weeks. For proximal pole fractures, operative reduction and fixation are indicated.[19]

Operative Repair

Operative reduction and internal fixation are indicated for unstable fracture patterns. Some authors advocate, however, that nondisplaced waist fractures should be treated operatively.[17,20] Rigid internal fixation may allow early mobilization, decrease time to union, and improve range of motion. A more rapid functional recovery and the potential for earlier to return to sports and work after operative repair are both appealing to many patients with nondisplaced scaphoid fractures. Cast immobilization does not eliminate micromotion at the fracture site and does not favorably alter the biologic environment to promote healing. McQueen and colleagues[21] in a prospective, randomized trial randomly allocated 60 consecutive patients with scaphoid waist fractures to percutaneous fixation with a cannulated Acutrak screw or cast immobilization. Patients who underwent percutaneous fixation showed a faster time to union and a more rapid return of function and return to sports with a low complication rate and work compared with those managed nonoperatively. A randomized, controlled trial and a recent meta-analysis have been done to compare surgery versus conservative management of undisplaced waist fractures.[17,20] The rate of complications in the surgical treatment groups was significant with small comparative treatment effect. The complications include infection, complex regional pain syndrome (CPRS), prominent hardware, technical difficulties intraoperatively, scar-related complications, scaphotrapeziotrapezoid joint osteoarthritis in surgical treatment group, and radiocarpal osteoarthritis in the nonoperative group.

Fixation Methods

A variety of implants have been examined to optimize the stabilization and healing of scaphoid fractures. Management and fixation constructs have to take into account the bone quality, fracture pattern, and reduction. The implant has to counter bending, shearing, and translational forces that act at the fracture site. Implants used for fixation include Kirschner (K)-wires, traditional screws placed in compression, headless compression screws, cannulated screws of both types, and bioabsorbable implants.

Studies have reported that cannulated screws have resulted in a higher rate of central placement in the scaphoid with better resistance and compressive forces. McCallister and colleagues[22] simulated scaphoid waist fractures and biomechanically compared screws placed in the central axis with screws placed eccentrically. Fixation with central placement of the screw demonstrated 43% greater stiffness, 113% greater load at 2 mm of displacement, and 39% greater load at failure. Trumble and colleagues,[23] found that screws should be placed centrally within the middle third of the proximal pole of the scaphoid on both the anterioposterior and lateral views in displaced scaphoid fractures.

Long, centrally placed screws (that end 2 to 3 mm under the chondral surface) offer superior biomechanical stability than short, eccentrically placed screws (**Fig. 6**). Longer screws reduce forces at the fracture site and spread bending forces along the screw. A screw placed centrally and deep in the cancellous bone of the scaphoid optimizes the stability conferred by scaphoid screw fixation.[5] However, one has to be careful with the length to avoid prominence at the chondral surface. In addition, it is critical to adequately ream the scaphoid central guide wire to obtain compression rather than distraction. Scaphoid screws should be no longer than 4 mm less than the measured scaphoid length (leaving ≥2 mm of bone coverage at both ends of the scaphoid). Screw prominence at the articular surface leads to unacceptable hardware impingement and subsequent chondral wear. When rigid fixation

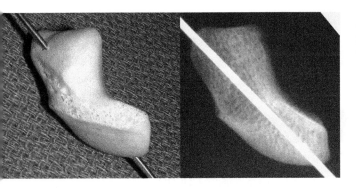

Fig. 6. Central pin placement. (*From* Slade JF, Merrell GA. Minimally invasive management of scaphoid fractures. Operat Tech Plast Reconstr Surg 2002;9(4):143–50; with permission.)

cannot be provided by a central screw placement alone (such as in proximal pole fractures and nonunions), augmentation may be necessary to prevent micromotion at the fracture site. Supplemental fixation is commonly applied from the distal scaphoid to the capitate using a 0.062-in K-wire or a mini-headless screw.[5]

Screw fixation, however, is not without its complications. Neighboring structures can be damaged. A cadaveric study found that the extensor digitorum communis, extensor indicis proprius, extensor pollicis longus, and the capsular insertion of the posterior interosseus nerve were at risk of injury.[22] Furthermore, the screw had protruded into the radioscaphoid joint in 2 cases. A retrospective review of 24 scaphoid fractures treated with dorsal percutaneous screw fixation included failure of a screw to capture the distal fragment and intraoperative breakage of a guide wire.[24]

OPERATIVE TECHNIQUE

Both volar and dorsal approaches are described. Studies have shown that both the volar and the dorsal approaches offered reliable results. No differences have been identified between the 2 groups in terms of union time and functional outcome, which included pain, range of motion, return to work, and grip strength. The choice of approach is dictated by the fracture location. The dorsal, antegrade approach is the preferred approach for proximal pole fractures, whereas a volar, retrograde approach may provide better fracture stability for distal pole fractures. Waist fractures are amenable to either approach.

Volar Open Approach

The open volar approach to the scaphoid requires a longitudinal incision, over the FCR tendon extended between the thenar muscles and the abductor pollicis longus tendon. This incision is carried proximally to 2 cm from the scaphoid

tuberosity. The distal incision is in line with the thumb metacarpal. The ulnar border of the FCR is avoided to minimize trauma to the palmar cutaneous branch of the median nerve. The FCR tendon sheath is divided and the tendon is retracted ulnar-ward. The pericapsular fat is divided and this exposes the wrist capsule. The long radiolunate and RSC ligaments are sharply divided, which exposes the scaphoid waist. When closing, attention to proper repair of the volar carpal ligaments must be met to avoid problems with iatrogenic carpal instability.

Volar Percutaneous Technique

A percutaneous technique may also be used to limit soft-tissue dissection and to protect the integrity of the volar carpal ligaments. In this technique, the STT joint is identified and marked on the volar side of the skin. A closed reduction is applied. A transverse stab incision is made at about 1 cm distal to the scaphotrapezial joint under image intensifier control. After blunt dissection to the distal end of the scaphoid, a 0.45-in K-wire is used for provisional reduction and stabilization along the long axis of the scaphoid and is directed (under fluoroscopic guidance) toward the center of the proximal pole. The length of the central guide wire within the scaphoid is determined. After hand reaming, a compression screw of appropriate length is advanced under fluoroscopy. The screw is buried to avoid intra-articular prominence (**Fig. 7**).

The Dorsal Open Approach

The open dorsal approach to the scaphoid provides better access to the proximal scaphoid. This approach, however, can be a concern because of injury to the vascular supply of the scaphoid. The advantage is better targeting of the central axis of the scaphoid and allowing more precise placement of the screw within the scaphoid. Furthermore, one avoids injury to the volar carpal ligaments protecting stability.

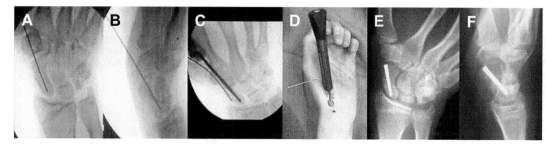

Fig. 7. Volar percutaneous technique. (*A, B*) Guidewire placement. (*C*) Drilling over guidewire. (*D*) Inserting screw. (*E, F*) Anterioposterior/lateral images of screw placement. (*From* Haisman JM, Rohde RS, Weiland AJ et al. Acute fractures of the scaphoid. J Bone Joint Surg Am 2006;88:2750–58.)

A longitudinal incision is made over the scapholunate interval and radiocarpal joint (**Fig. 8**). The skin flaps are elevated and care is taken to protect the radial sensory nerve. The EPL is identified and retracted radially. The septum between the third and fourth compartments is opened and the extensor tendons are retracted ulnar-ward. The capsule is incised radial to the border of the dorsal radiocarpal ligament. With this approach, the entire proximal two thirds of the scaphoid, the radial styloid, and the scaphoid fossa in the distal radius can be exposed.

Dorsal Percutaneous Technique

The open approach to fixation risk violating carpal ligaments with risk of carpal instability and potentially violating the blood supply; thus, there is an increasing trend to toward percutaneous fixation of scaphoid fractures, both displaced and undisplaced. Percutaneous technique allows for less soft-tissue dissection and subsequent faster healing.

The patient is placed supine and the hand is outstretched on a hand table. Landmarks are drawn on the pronated wrist. Under appropriate anesthesia with the patient in a supine position, the dorsal scapholunate interval is marked. Scaphoid reduction is assessed fluoroscopically. K-wires (usually 0.062") can be placed in the distal and proximal poles of the scaphoid and can be used as joysticks for manipulative reduction of a displaced fracture. The wrist is pronated and flexed until the scaphoid is seen as a circle on fluoroscopy. The center of the circle is chosen as the target point for the insertion of the guide wire into the proximal pole of the scaphoid. A small longitudinal skin incision is made over the center of the circle, soft tissues are dissected bluntly to the joint capsule, and a percutaneous arthrotomy is made with a small blunt tipped hemostat. The guide wire is driven dorsal to volar in an antegrade fashion so that it exits at the radial base of the

thumb. The reduction and central placement of the guide wire is confirmed under fluoroscopy. A pilot hole is drilled along the guide K-wire. After tapping, a headless screw is inserted under fluoroscopy in a freehand manner (**Fig. 9**).

ARTHROSCOPIC-ASSISTED PERCUTANEOUS SCAPHOID FRACTURE REPAIR

Arthroscopy can also be used to help with diagnosis of concurrent ligamentous injury such as the triangular fibrocartiligous complex and as a way to judge reduction of the fracture (**Fig. 10**). For example, midcarpal arthroscopy enables direct visualization of the articular reduction of a scaphoid waist fracture along the scaphocapitate articulation. An important tip is to place the central scaphoid osseus wire to prevent any displacement during the athroscopic assessment.[24]

Bone Loss Acute Fractures

Bone defects can occur with scaphoid fractures and the amount of defect depends on the fracture location, as well as the degree of comminution. A highly comminuted fracture presents technical difficulty in that screw purchase may be challenging. One has to be ready to have options such as traditional K wire fixation or even nonoperative treatment. CT in these instances are very useful to determine the amount of bone loss and to help to delineate the fracture management and subsequent appropriate management.

Malunion, Delayed Union, and Nonunion

Many variables influence treatment of a malunion, delayed union, or nounion: Previous treatment and duration, patient's activity and personal demands, as well as the surgeon's preference.

Oka and colleagues[25] looked at bone defects in scaphoid nonunion and found that the both the shape and amount of the defect differed with the fracture type. In distal fractures, a humpback deformity is seen and the bone defect is large

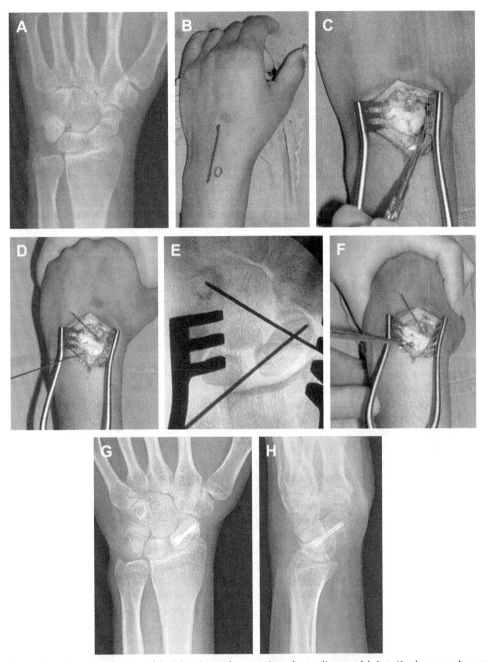

Fig. 8. Open dorsal approach. Dorsal incision is made exposing the radiocarpal joint. K-wires may be used for distal pole control as well as for provisional stabilization. (*From* Kawamura K, Chung KC. Treatment of scaphoid fractures and nonunions. J Hand Surg Am 2008;33(6):988–97; with permission.)

and triangular. Proximal fractures tend to have smaller defects with crescent-shaped patterns. The finding of this study suggested that both the pattern and amount of bone loss had to do with location of the fracture line relative to the dorsal apex of the scaphoid ridge. This is where the dorsal component of the scapholunate (SL) ligament and proximal part of the dorsal intercarpal

ligament are located. They both provide stability to the dorsal scaphoid. In the distal fractures, the fracture line goes beyond these ligamentous attachments, which cause an inability of the fragment to resist flexion forces, resulting in the humpback deformity. In the proximal fractures, the ligaments remain attached on the distal fragment providing stability.

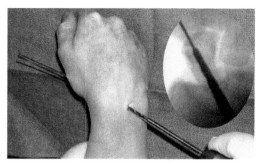

Fig. 9. Dorsal percutaneous technique. (*From* Slade JF, Merrell GA. Minimally invasive management of scaphoid fractures. Operat Tech Plast Reconstr Surg 2002;9(4):143–50; with permission.)

Type of Bone Graft

The gold standard has typically been to use iliac crest bone in the treatment of scaphoid fracture. This was owing to the supposed superior biomechanical strength and osteogenic capacity. However, other sources such as the distal radius are viable sources of autogenous bone graft.

The studies that have compared these graft options have shown that the union rates were similar with both techniques. Tambe and colleagues[26] have documented 66% and 67% graft union in nonunited scaphoids treated by iliac crest bone graft and distal radius bone graft, respectively. There is also increased morbidity with the use of the iliac crest bone such has pain, infection, hematoma, and injury to the lateral femoral cutaneous nerve. This suggests the distal radius is an improved alternative given it only involves a minor increase in surgical exposure.[26]

The authors' preferred method is to use iliac crest bone graft. It has long been considered the gold standard for autogenous bone graft source with proven biomechanical strength and osteogenic capacity.

Nonunions

Nonunion rates range from 5% to 25% (**Fig. 11**).[8,9,14,26,27] Factors that increase the risk are displacement of more than 1 mm, fracture of the proximal pole, history of osteonecrosis, vertical oblique fracture pattern, and nicotine use.[8,9,14,26,27] Nonunion can result in pain, altered carpal kinematics, and decreased range of motion, leading to disuse osteoporosis, weakness in grip, and degenerative arthritis. For an established symptomatic nonunion, whether it is fibrous or sclerotic, it should be treated with open repair and bone grafting. Proximal pole nonunion are best visualized through a dorsal approach and waist fractures should be managed by an approach that allows for a volarly placed bone graft. A humpback deformity requires an open approach with reduction of the scaphoid alignment and a corticocancellous wedge graft.

For conventional bone grafting of scaphoid nonunions, a recent study concluded that union rates were affected adversely by manual labor, nonunions of more than 5 years' duration, concomitant radial styloidectomy, and inadequate duration of postoperative immobilization.[28] Inoue and Kuwahata[28] reported that failure of conventional bone grafting with screw fixation of scaphoid nonunions was related to the existence of AVN of the proximal fragment, instability of the fracture fragment, prolonged delay in surgery, and fracture location.

Excision of the scaphoid distal pole can be used for nonunion of the scaphoid without advanced degenerative change. Ruch and colleagues[19,29–31] reported good results after arthroscopic excision of the distal pole for the treatment of AVN of the proximal pole. Malerich and colleagues[32] described this technique for the treatment of SNAC wrist. After removal of the scaphoid distal pole, carpal loads are transferred primarily to the radius through the radiolunate articulation (**Fig. 12**). There is a theoretic concern that degenerative changes

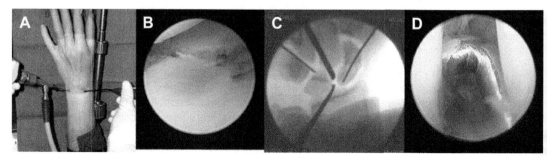

Fig. 10. The thumb is suspended from the traction tower, which allows switching from the AP to lateral projections when placing the guidewire. (*From* Slade JF, Merrell GA. Minimally invasive management of scaphoid fractures. Operat Tech Plast Reconstr Surg 2002;9(4):143–50; with permission.)

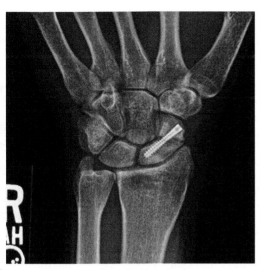

Fig. 11. Nonunion of scaphoid waist fracture.

in the radiolunate joint can occur; however, studies have not demonstrated this equivocally.

Nonvascularized Bone Grafting

Nonvascularized bone grafting is probably sufficient for most waist fracture nonunions without AVN. Cases of proximal pole AVN, a failed previous surgery, or long duration of the nonunion should be considered for vascularized bone graft. Stark and colleagues reported successful union in 97% of 151 scaphoid nonunions, and recently Finsen and colleagues[33] demonstrated success

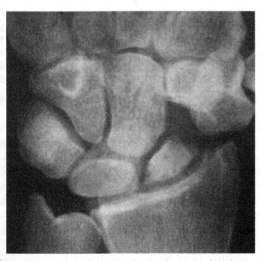

Fig. 12. Excision of the distal pole. (*From* Malerich MM, Clifford J, Eaton B, et al. Distal scaphoid resection arthroplasty for the treatment of degenerative arthritis secondary to scaphoid nonunion. J Hand Surg Am 1999;24:1196–205; with permission.)

in 90% of 39 nonunions with this technique. Notably, the results were also excellent for proximal pole nonunions in both studies. A corticocancellous wedge bone graft is inserted volarly at the nonunion site and the nonunion is repaired with either K-wires or screws. It can be difficult to shape the wedge graft accurately; hence, Stark offered an alternative technique to fix humpback deformities with nonunion, using temporary K-wire fixation and cancellous grafting.

Vascularized Bone Grafting

Vascularized bone grafting is used in many cases of nonunion, especially with cases of suspected or established AVN. Types of grafts include the pronator quadratus pedicled bone graft, or the palmar carpal artery, the radial styloid fasciosteal graft, and pedicled grafts from the index finger metacarpal and the thumb metacarpal. Zaidemberg described vascularized bone graft derived from the dorsal radial aspect of the distal radius, which is nourished by the 1,2 intercompartmental supraretinacular artery (1,2 ICSRA).[34] Free vascularized bone grafts from the iliac crest and the medial femoral supracondylar region have also been reported. Shin described a technique to harvest the medial femoral condyle bone graft based on the descending genicular artery or superomedial genicular artery.[35] Dissection and microvascular anastomosis of the vessel can be technically demanding and the need for pedicle rotation in some of those grafts may compromise the long-term patency. Sotereanos and colleagues[36] proposed the use of a vascularized bone graft that is capsular based. It is derived from the distal aspect of the distal radius and ulnar/distal to Listers tubercle. The advantage of this graft is its close proximity to the nonunion site without the need for excessive rotation. The vascular supply is derived from the strip of the dorsal capsule; a specific pedicle does not need to be dissected. One limitation of this technique includes the inability to correct a humpback deformity; in fact, an ideal indication for a dorsal capsular graft is a proximal pole nonunion. Another limitation is in patients who have had previous surgery or injury to the dorsal aspect of the wrist, because the vascularity of the capsule in those patients would not be predictable.

The principal advantage of vascularized bone grafting is a potentially more reliable union after grafting. A recent meta-analysis found that vascularized bone grafting achieved an 88% union rate compared with a 47% union rate with screw and intercalated wedge fixation in scaphoid nonunions with AVN.[37] Perlik and Guildford reported that increased density on the preoperative radiographs has only 40% accuracy for detecting proximal fragment avascularity, and thus many cases that were classified as AVN may actually have had satisfactory vascularity of the proximal pole.[38] Absence of punctuate bleeding from the proximal pole at surgery is a more accurate way of determining vascularity.

Boyer found a 60% healing rate in the study scaphoid nonunions treated by 1,2-ICSRA pedicled vascularized bone grafting.[39] All subjects in this study, however, had proximal pole AVN. Straw and colleagues[40] also reported only 2 of 16 nonunions with AVN united with the 1,2 ICSRA bone graft. Chang and colleagues[7] evaluated a large series of 1,2 ICSRA bone grafts that were performed for scaphoid nonunions and showed that 71% of 48 nonunions healed and the union rate was 91% in the absence of AVN and 63% in the presence of AVN. Successful outcome is not universal and depends on debridement of the nonunion site, reduction of scaphoid alignment, appropriate bone grafting, and rigid internal fixation, even when vascularized bone grafting is used for scaphoid nonunions.

Associated Instability

The scaphoid functions as a complex link between the proximal and distal carpal rows of the wrist. A scaphoid fracture nonunion changes wrist mechanics, which can lead to carpal instability and secondary degenerative changes. A high incidence of SL ligament injuries found in scaphoid nonunions has raised the possibility of an association between the 2 injuries.[11] This association raises the indication for arthroscopy even in nondisplaced scaphoid fractures if surgical fixation and early mobilization is offered to avoid detrimental effects of an undiagnosed ligament tear. The advantage of arthroscopy is direct evaluation of associated ligament injuries not seen in standard imaging, and it helps to confirm both fracture reduction and the absence of screw protrusion after osteosynthesis.

Pediatric Scaphoid Fractures

Scaphoid fractures are rare, as are most carpal fractures in children. The incidence is about 0.45% of all upper limb injuries in children and occurs typically in the teenage years.[41] In children, the ossification center is protected by a thick layer of cartilage, which accounts for the low incidence of fracture. As the ossification center changes with age, the pattern of injury also changes. Distal pole scaphoid fractures are more common in children as ossification progresses in a distal to proximal

direction.[41] As the child approaches adolescence, the fracture pattern becomes similar to that in adults.

When examining the patient, it is important to have a high index of suspicion. Given the rarity of this fracture in children and difficulties with interpreting radiographs of a pediatric carpus, a scaphoid fracture can be missed. When interpreting radiographs, one should also be aware that the distance from the ossified lunate and scaphoid decreases as the child approaches adolescence. This is a normal radiographic finding, which changes with the age of the child. As the proximal pole matures and ossifies, the average scapholunate interval is 9 mm in a 7-year-old and 3 mm in a 15-year-old.

Management of most pediatric scaphoid fractures is with cast immobilization. Given that most are distal pole fractures (60%–85%), excellent healing is reported. Furthermore, most pediatric scaphoid fractures are nondisplaced or involve only 1 cortex. Proximal pole fractures are rare. For avulsion and incomplete fractures, a short thumb spica cast is recommended for 6 weeks. In the younger child, a long arm cast may be appropriate to prevent the cast from falling off. For waist and transverse fractures, 8 weeks of immobilization is recommended. It is reasonable to confirm healing with a CT scan before return to activity for a patient treated nonoperatively in a cast.

Nonunion of scaphoid fractures is a rare occurrence in children. Delayed presentation or failure of initial diagnosis contributes to nonunion. Most scaphoid nonunions in skeletally immature patients involve the scaphoid waist. Mintzer reported a series of 13 scaphoid nonunions in children ages 9 to 15 years. These fractures were treated with surgical stabilization and all healed.[42]

Fabre and De Boeck reviewed the literature and reported that of 371 children with acute scaphoid fracture treated with immobilization, only 3 (0.8%) developed a nonunion.[43] They found only 29 published cases of scaphoid nonunion in children. In their own series of 23 acute fractures of the scaphoid in children, all healed with cast immobilization. They also reported 2 cases of patients who had scaphoid nonunion that presented late after their injuries (referred from other institutions) at an average of 7 to 11 months after their injuries. Both were treated successfully with cast immobilization.

Another large series of scaphoid fractures (64 cases) reported 46 nonunions.[41] All the nonunion cases were waist fractures, except for 1 proximal and 1 distal pole fracture. The patients were between 11 and 15 years of age, and most injuries resented late. The reasons for delayed presentation were reluctance to forgo play on teams or report the injury, and symptoms that were not severe enough to warrant expedient evaluation.

COST ANALYSIS

There continues to be cost analysis debate regarding both the role of surgery versus casting in the management of undisplaced or minimally displaced waist and distal pole scaphoid fractures. Both casting and surgery are reliable treatments and outcomes are comparable. Davis and colleagues[44] performed a cost-utility analysis of open reduction and internal fixation versus cast immobilization for acute nondisplaced midwaist scaphoid fractures. They concluded that open reduction and internal fixation offered more quality-adjusted life-years and is less costly than casting ($7940 vs $13,851 per patient) because of a longer period of lost productivity with casting.[13] When only considering direct costs incurred by Medicare reimbursement, casting was less costly than open reduction and internal fixation ($605 vs $1747). The authors did state, however, that the cost-utility analysis overestimates lost productivity with casting because people in casts can still work.

Vinnars[45–47] found that the total hospital costs were lower with cast treatment than surgery. They also found that manual laborers had a longer time off of work, especially if they received casting alone. They did not find the same difference with casting in nonmanual workers. The decision to operate versus casting depends on the individual's unique circumstances. Surgery is more expensive in the initial period; however, allowing an individual to get back to work faster may ultimately incur less costs with respect to workers compensation. Ultimately, if an individual's employment is hand and upper extremity intensive, surgery ultimately may be the more cost-effective management.

REFERENCES

1. Bohler L, Trojan E, Jahna H. The results of treatment of 734 fresh, simple fractures of the scaphoid. J Hand Surg Br 2003;28:319–31.
2. Van Tassel DC, Owens BD, Wolf JM. Incidence estimates and demographics of scaphoid fracture in the US population. J Hand Surg Am 2010;35:1242–5.
3. Wolf JM, Dawson L, Mountcastle SB, et al. The incidence of scaphoid fracture in a military population. Injury 2009;40:1316–9.
4. Heinzelmann AD, Archer G, Bindra RR. Anthropmetry of the human scaphoid. J Hand Surg Am 2007; 32A:988–97.
5. Dodds SD, Panjabi MM, Slade JF. Screw fixation of scaphoid fractures: a biomechanical assessment of screw length and screw augmentation. J Hand Surg Am 2006;31:405–13.
6. Bindra RR. Scaphoid density by CT scan. Bucharest (Hungary): IFSSH; 2004.
7. Chang MA, Bishop AT, Moran SL, et al. The outcomes and complications of 1.2 intercompartmental supraretinacular artery pedicled vascularized bone grafting of scaphoid nonunions. J Hand Surg Am 2006;31:387–96.
8. Jones DB, Burger H, Bishop AT, et al. Treatment of scaphoid waist nonunions with an avascular proximal pole and carpal collapse. A comparison of two vascularized bone grafts. J Bone Joint Surg Am 2008;90:2616–25.
9. Kawamura K, Chung K. Treatment of scaphoid fractures and nonunions. J Hand Surg Am 2008; 33:988–97.
10. Buijze GA, Lozano-Calderon SA, Strackee SD, et al. Osseus and ligamentous scaphoid anatomy: part 1. A systematic literature review highlighting controversies. J Hand Surg Am 2011;36:1926–35.
11. Jorgsholm P, Thomse NO, Bjorkman A, et al. The incidence of intrinsic and extrinsic ligament injuries in scaphoid waist fractures. J Hand Surg Am 2010; 35:368–74.
12. Adey L, Souer JS, Lozano-Calderon S, et al. Computed tomography of suspected scaphoid fractures. J Hand Surg Am 2007;32:61–6.
13. Buijze A, Doornberg JN, Ham JS, et al. Surgical compared with conservative treatment for acute nondisplaced or minimally displaced scaphoid fractures, a systematic review and meta analysis of randomized controlled trials. J Bone Joint Surg Am 2010;92:1534–44.
14. Moritomo H, Murase T, Kunihiro O, et al. Relationship between the fracture and location and the kinematic pattern in scaphoid nonunion. J Hand Surg Am 2008;33:1459–68.
15. Wolfe SW, Neu C, Crisco JJ. In vivo scaphoid, lunate, and capitate kinematics in flexion and extension. J Hand Surg Am 2000;25A:860–89.
16. Mallee W, Doornber JN, Ring D, et al. Comparison of CT and MRI for diagnosis of suspected scaphoid fractures. J Bone Joint Surg Am 2011;93:20–8.
17. Ibrahim T, Oureshi A, Sutton AJ, et al. Surgical versus nonsurgical treatment of acute minimally displaced and undisplaced scaphoid waist fractures: pairwise and network meta-analyses of randomized controlled trials. J Hand Surg Am 2011;36:1759–68.
18. Pillai A, Jain M. Management of clinical fractures of the scaphoid: results of an audit and literature review. Eur J Emerg Med 2005;12(2):47–51.
19. Ram AN, Chung KC. Evidence-based management of acute nondisplaced scaphoid waist fractures. J Hand Surg Am 2009;34:734–78.

20. Vinnars B, Pietreanu M, Bodestedt A, et al. Nonoperative compared with operative treatment of acute scaphoid fractures, a randomized clinical trial. J Bone Joint Surg Am 2008;90:1176–85.

21. McQueen MM, Gelbke MK, Wakefield A, et al. Percutaneous screw fixation versus conservative treatment for fractures of the waist of the scaphoid: a prospective randomized study. J Bone Joint Surg Br 2008;90:66–71.

22. McCallister WV, Knight J, Kaliappan R, et al. Central placement of the screw in simulated fractures of the scaphoid waist: a biomechanical study. J Bone Joint Surg Am 2003;85-A(1):72–7.

23. Trumble TE, Gilbert M, Murray LW, et al. Displaced scaphoid fractures treated with open reduction and internal fixation with a cannulated screw. J Bone Joint Surg Am 2000;82(5):633–41.

24. Leon IH, Micic ID, Oh CW, et al. Percutaneous screw fixation for scaphoid fracture: a comparison between dorsal and volar approaches. J Hand Surg Am 2009; 34:228–36.

25. Oka K, Murase T, Moritomo H, et al. Patterns of bone defect in scaphoid non-union: a 3 dimensional and quantitative analysis. J Hand Surg Am 2005;30: 359–65.

26. Jarrett P, Kinzel V, Stoffel K. A biomechanical comparison of scaphoid fixation with bone grafting using iliac bone or distal radius bone. J Hand Surg Am 2007;32:1367–73.

27. Wong K, Von Schroeder HP. Delays and poor management of scaphoid fractures: factors contributing to nonunion. J Hand Surg Am 2011;36: 1471–4.

28. Inoue G, Kuwahata Y. Repeat screw stabilization with bone grafting after a failed Herbert screw fixation for acute scaphoid fracture nonunions. J Hand Surg Am 1997;22:413–48.

29. Leventhal EL, Wolfe SW, Moore DC, et al. Interfragmentary motion in patients with scaphoid nonunion. J Hand Surg Am 2008;33:1108–15.

30. Ruch DS, Papadonikolakis A. Resection of the scaphoid distal pole for symptomatic scaphoid nonunion after failed previous surgical treatment. J Hand Surg Am 2006;31:588–93.

31. Payatakes A, Sotereanos DG. Pedicles vascularized bone grafts for scaphoid and lunate reconstruction. J Am Acad Orthop Surg 2009;17:744–55.

32. Vance MC, Catalano LW, Malerich MM. Distal scaphoid resection for arthritis secondary to scaphoid nonunion: a twenty year experience: level 4 evidence. J Hand Surg Am 2011;36(Suppl).

33. Stark HH, Rickard TA, Zemel NP, et al. Treatment of ununited fractures of the scaphoid by iliac bone grafts and Kirschner-wire fixation. J Bone Joint Surg Am 1998;70A:982–91.

34. Zaidemberg C, Siebert JW, Angrigiani C. A new vascularized bone graft for scaphoid nonunion. J Hand Surg Am 1991;16A:474–8.

35. Sammer DM, Bishop AT, Shin AY. Vascularized medial femoral condyle graft for thumb metacarpal reconstruction: case report. J Hand Surg Am 2009 34:715–78.

36. Sotereanos DG, Darlis NA, Dailiana ZH, et al. A capsular based vascularized distal radius graft for proximal pole scaphoid pseudarthrosis. J Hand Surg Am 2006;31:580–7.

37. Merrell GA, Wolfe SW, Slade JF. Treatment of scaphoid nonunions: quantitative meta-analysis of the literature. J Hand Surg Am 2002;27:685–91.

38. Perlik PC, Guilford WB. Magnetic resonance imaging to assess vascularity of scaphoid nonunions. J Hand Surg Am 1991;16A:479–84.

39. Boyer MI, Von Schroeder HP, Axelrod TS. Scaphoid nonunion with avascular necrosis of the proximal pole: treatment with a vascularized bone graft from the dorsum of the distal radius. J Hand Surg B 1998;23B:686–90.

40. Straw RG, Davis TR, Dias JJ. Scaphoid nonunion (treatment with vascularized bone graft based on the 1,2 –intercompartmental supraretinacular branch of the radial artery). J Hand Surg Br 2002;27B:413–46.

41. Gholson JJ, Bae DS, Zurakowski D, et al. Scaphoid fractures in children and adolescents: contemporary injury patterns and factors influencing time to union. J Bone Joint Surg Am 2011;93:1210–29.

42. Mintzer CM, Waters PM. Surgical treatment of pediatric scaphoid fracture nonunions. J Pediatr Orthop 1999;19:236–9.

43. Fabre O, De Boeck H, Haentiens P. Fractures and nonunions of the carpal scaphoid in children. Acta Orthop Belg 2001;67:121–5.

44. Davis E, Chung K, Kotsis S, et al. A cost/utility analysis of open reduction and internal fixation versus cast immobilization for acute non-displaced mid waist scaphoid fractures. Plast Reconstr Surg 2006;117:1223–35.

45. Vinnars B. Scaphoid fractures: studies on diagnosis and treatment, digital comprehensive summaries of Uppsala dissertations. 2008:11–35.

46. Waitayawinyu T, McCallister WV, Nemechek NM et al. Surgical techniques: scaphoid nonunion. J Am Acad Orthop Surg 2007;15:308–20.

47. Brooks S, Cicuttini FM, Lim S, et al. Cost effectiveness of adding magnetic resonance imaging to the usual management of suspected scaphoid fractures. Br J Sports Med 2005;39(2):75–9.

Index

Note: Page numbers of article titles are in **boldface** type.

Orthop Clin N Am 44 (2013) 121–123
http://dx.doi.org/10.1016/S0030-5898(12)00126-5

orthopedic.theclinics.com

Moving?

Make sure your subscription moves with you!

To notify us of your new address, find your **Clinics Account Number** (located on your mailing label above your name), and contact customer service at:

Email: journalscustomerservice-usa@elsevier.com

800-654-2452 (subscribers in the U.S. & Canada)
314-447-8871 (subscribers outside of the U.S. & Canada)

Fax number: 314-447-8029

Elsevier Health Sciences Division
Subscription Customer Service
3251 Riverport Lane
Maryland Heights, MO 63043

*To ensure uninterrupted delivery of your subscription, please notify us at least 4 weeks in advance of move.

ELSEVIER

Printed and bound by CPI Group (UK) Ltd, Croydon, CR0 4YY

03/10/2024

01040344-0006